ENDOMETRIOSIS IN PRIMARY CARE

The burden of endometriosis is enormous, with one in ten women suffering from this painful and debilitating condition. It is estimated to affect 1.5 million women in the UK and 190 million women globally. Despite its prevalence, it is currently taking an average of eight years for women to receive a formal diagnosis, with 27 being the average age at which a diagnosis is made. This can have a significant impact on the physical and mental health of those living with the condition, with 30–40% experiencing infertility.

An early, accurate diagnosis in a primary care setting can have a crucial impact on the care a patient with endometriosis receives, providing the opportunity for prompt referral, advice on managing the condition and connecting the sufferer with wider support networks. This timely, practical book brings together clear and concise information for GPs and primary health care teams on how this can be achieved quickly, accurately and effectively.

ENDOMETRIOSIS IN PRIMARY CARE

A Practical Guide

Anita Sharma

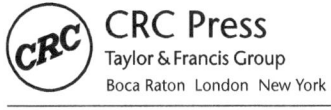

CRC Press
Taylor & Francis Group
Boca Raton London New York

CRC Press is an imprint of the
Taylor & Francis Group, an **informa** business

Designed cover images: With thanks to Anbreen Latif, Caitlin Leah Banks, Claire Warburton, Courtney Ormrod, Emma Wareing, Jo Walton, Lorna Marsh, Lucy Bowker, Rachael Pennington and Rebecca Lomas (front cover) and to Cohen J. Loveder, Deborah P. Fischer, Kay Marshall and Catherine E.W. Pennington (back cover, from left to right).

First edition published 2025
by CRC Press
2385 NW Executive Center Drive, Suite 320, Boca Raton FL 33431

and by CRC Press
4 Park Square, Milton Park, Abingdon, Oxon, OX14 4RN

CRC Press is an imprint of Taylor & Francis Group, LLC

ISBN: 978-1-032-68480-2 (hbk)
ISBN: 978-1-032-68479-6 (pbk)
ISBN: 978-1-032-68481-9 (ebk)

DOI: 10.1201/9781032684819

Typeset in Sabon
by Apex CoVantage, LLC

Access the support materials: www.routledge.com/9781032684796

Contents

For Patient Information Leaflet Sample *see eResource*: www.routledge.com/9781032684796
(Copyright Northern Care Alliance NHS Foundation Trust. Made available with permission.)

Foreword

By Gaity Ahmad

I met Dr Sharma when our roads crossed through her charity work with Endometriosis Awareness North. Her background as a general practitioner, hard work and interest in the patients affected by the condition puts her in a perfect position to put together this book.

This book is a way to bring together the latest information on what endometriosis is, how it is investigated and diagnosed, current management and what the current research field is working on to improve the lives of our patients, their families and for society as a whole.

Working as a consultant gynaecologist in minimal access laparoscopic gynaecological surgery within the Northern Care Alliance (NCA) NHS Trusts, I have come across many patients, each with their own journey in managing their symptoms and disease. It is not infrequent that they describe the lack of understanding of their symptoms and the condition by health care professionals and wider society. Aiming this book at different roles amongst health care professionals will hopefully help bridge this gap in knowledge and understanding of the complexity of managing these patients.

I hope you enjoy the chapter on surgical management of endometriosis, which I have co-authored. Hopefully, it will give you an insight into the current surgical management guidelines. We are fortunate and proud within NCA to work in a British Society of Gynaecological Endoscopy (BSGE)–accredited endometriosis centre with a full multidisciplinary team to provide safe-care with the aim to keep our patients in the centre of our mission.

Miss Gaity Ahmad MBBS MD MSc FRCOG
Clinical Director for Gynaecology at Oldham/Rochdale/Fairfield
Clinical Lead for the Northern Care Alliance Endometriosis Centre
Honorary Senior Lecturer at Manchester University

Foreword

By Peter Gibson

There are those who will ponder the irony of a book around endometriosis beginning with a recommendation from a male. As this foreword and indeed the rest of this tome will reveal, those identifying as such have little or no understanding of the condition unless it affects their family or social unit, directly. At this time of rabid gender politics, the charge I am about to make may also appear incendiary. But the reason Dr Anita Sharma has penned this polemic on endometriosis is because men have too often dismissed or discarded a condition that affects one-in-ten women of childbearing age and remained blissfully aware of the pain some of their sisters (or indeed anyone with a uterus) might suffer.

I once numbered myself in the second bracket, being aware of, but not invested in solving, the condition of endometriosis. It took Dr Sharma's influence, and the experience of the case studies she introduced me to, for that to actually change. And that is the hope with this book, that it enlightens those amongst the populace who are ignorant and pricks the conscience of decision-makers, health chiefs and medics to do more to research, diagnose with more alacrity and even find a cure for a condition which one woman recently described as, "like having cement in your stomach."

Dr Sharma's powers of persuasion have spanned across a career in general practice, and she has sometimes been a lone voice in advocating essential change in the male-dominated sphere of health care. From passionate pleas for more pessary clinics to calls for greater expertise at the primary care level to treat men's mental health, her sometimes gentle, always thoughtful and more than occasionally highly moral challenge has improved patient care for the better. Possessing a unique rapport with all, one of her prime achievements has been to bring communities from a great diaspora of backgrounds together, in the name of compassion. No mean feat in this divisive age. Little wonder, then, that she plays such a prominent role in organizations such as National Institute for Care Excellence (NICE) and British International Doctors Association (BIDA), leads local charitable concerns such as the Inner Wheel (Rochdale) and is so actively involved in assessing and encouraging the next generation of general practitioners.

One of the most important facets of leadership, though, is knowing when to step back. Allow others to further your cause. And I am sure Dr Sharma will forgive me for saying that when it comes to engendering change around endometriosis, it is the patient's experience that is the most effective.

She has opened the pages of this book to Lucy Bowker and Courtney Ormrod, who, when they relay the reality of lives blighted by endometriosis, have the power to move. This has been witnessed at events where they have spoken and staged at the likes of the University of Central Lancashire School of Medicine and in front of elected mayors and others of political influence. It is no exaggeration to say that their testimony frequently leads to tears.

Both bright and brave, their ambassadorial roles for Dr Sharma's fledgling charity Endometriosis Awareness North have been encouraged and supported by those who love them most. And Courtney and Lucy have brought forward their families to share the impact of endometriosis on them, too. Both have fathers that served in blue light emergency services who have used their contacts to put the charity in front of the Greater Manchester Police officers, promoting a culture of endometriosis awareness within forces. The fact that they are male is also powerful emblematically; being a reminder that solving the issue is societal and not just a "woman's problem."

During the short life span of Dr Sharma's charity, commissioned surveys have revealed just how far we need to travel to reach our goals. Public perception of the condition is so poor that some respondents told us they thought endometriosis was a throat infection! But what was really disturbing was the dearth of knowledge within the medical profession, a fact echoed by our many case studies. Endometriosis is ill-researched. Diagnosis, slow and painful. Dire current resources means specialist services are not available. Time constraints have endometriosis sufferers leaving A&E units simply armed with purely paracetamol for back pain. Lack of open-mindedness results in patients dismissed because they are too young or old to match the archetypal sufferer. And, most tragically of all, misogyny, stigma and prejudice play their part in pushing the condition to the margins.

To spark change, Dr Sharma has involved the charity in places where speaking about gynaecology is shunned. Her work in bringing together religious and cultural communities (the South Asian population in Oldham, particularly) has been commendable. Giving them a place to communicate openly and then feeding back to medical decision-makers has been pivotal. It is my hope that those who work within all spheres of health care use this book as an inspiration, an agent of change, and take its constructive criticism in that usual and commendable spirit of learning and change that rightly places the medical profession in such high regard. We are, and should be, forever learning.

I began this foreword by confessing that I knew little about endometriosis prior to my encounter with Dr Sharma. Since then, she has opened my eyes to the fact that endometriosis is merely part of a general malaise usually labelled "health inequalities." Statistics show that whilst there has been an increase in life expectancy for men, mortality rates for females have stagnated. The fact that COVID-19 struck more vehemently in disadvantaged communities proved starkly the need to provide decent health care services for all, regardless of gender, age, culture and class.

Such inequity is demonstrable within the South Asian community in Greater Manchester. Dr Sharma has used her influence to address women at pivotal projects such as CHAI Oldham and campaigned for greater openness within this and other marginalized communities. There are occasions where gynaecological issues are seen as taboo and decisions made (particularly when appointment letters for women drop though the door) by others and often without consultation with medics. Added to the aforementioned societal misogyny, poorer health services and living conditions, even air quality and lack of nutritional food creates just the kind of discrepancy in quality of life Dr Sharma talks about.

One last point of ignorance before you embark upon what I hope will be your endometriosis voyage of discovery. I certainly didn't equate endometriosis with such levels of despair until Endometriosis Awareness North conducted their first survey on the link between the condition and wellbeing. Weariness, certainly. Anxiety, definitely. But hopelessness and even dark thoughts? This is shameful and the inability to recognize the condition and administer appropriate care has surely played a part.

I see it as no coincidence that since Dr Sharma founded her charity, the entire profile of endometriosis has risen. That has involved celebrities coming forward, including broadcaster Naga Munchetty, and relaying their personal struggles with the condition. Internationally, country singer and film actor Dolly Parton revealed her battles with both the physical and mental aspects of endometriosis.

That was back in the 1980s.

The pace of change around this condition has been pitiful, but the seeds have been sown to tackle both the treatment of endometriosis and indeed many of the female health conditions so tragically ignored. Some of that is directly down to Dr Anita Sharma, but she would be the first to admit she cannot achieve this alone.

So, read the book, invest in its medical knowledge, case studies and recommendations and truly support the battle to support our sisters and reduce health inequalities.

Peter Gibson
Founder and Executive Director of PeteGibsonMedia

Foreword

Members of my research team were pleased to be given the opportunity, by Dr Sharma, to contribute to this book and to make a contribution to raising awareness of the multifaceted disease that is endometriosis. I have also had the pleasure of contributing to an event organized by Dr Sharma during which two young women explained how endometriosis had impacted them and their families. As a researcher, I know quite a lot about endometriosis at a cellular level, and it is very easy to get submerged in mediators and mechanisms and, in doing so, lose sight of what is happening to the whole person. Listening to women recounting what had and was happening to them made a marked impression on me and whenever things don't go as well as I would have wished in the laboratory, I take my mind back to those moving testimonials, and it spurs me on to keep going.

There are many definitions of what an unmet medical need (UMN) is, and they are similar to the one cited by the European Commission in 2006 of "a condition for which there exists no satisfactory method of diagnosis, prevention or treatment authorized in the Community or, even if such a method exists, in relation to which the medicinal product concerned will be of major therapeutic advantage to those affected." Some descriptions also reference societal need to encompass disease-related expenditure, epidemiology and psychosocial wellbeing. As you read through this book, you will become aware that endometriosis does indeed have all the characteristics of an unmet medical need and that we need to do more to produce more effective therapeutics which work without damaging fertility.

I hope you enjoy reading this book and that it gives you some insight into this rapidly evolving research field.

Kay Marshall BPharm PhD MBA FHEA FRPharmS FPhS
Professor of Reproductive Endocrine Pharmacology
University of Manchester

Preface

National Institute for Health and Clinical Excellence (NICE) quality standards are being developed to make it clear to service providers what quality care means. The quality standards are a set of specific, concise statements that are based on best available evidence and act as markers of high-quality, cost-effective patient care. As a GP with a special interest in gynaecology, women's health stands high on my agenda in order to both provide and maintain effective and evidenced-based management.

Women's health has, in my opinion, always been ignored due to the absence of a Quality Outcome Framework (QOF) in any of the gynaecological areas. In July 2022, the Women's Health Strategy for England was published. The ten-year ambition of the strategy includes measures to reduce lengthy diagnosis times, improve care for those with endometriosis, as well as provide more support for health care professionals and increased funding for research.

Endometriosis, a chronic inflammatory gynaecological disease marked by the presence of endometrial-like tissue outside the uterus, is estimated to affect 1.5 million women in the UK and 190 million women worldwide. It has significant social, public health and economic implications.

Under recognition, poor understanding and delayed treatment of this condition leave many women feeling unsupported. The annual health care burden of endometriosis in the UK is £12.5 billion in treatment and work loss.

Almost 60% of women will see three or more clinicians before a diagnosis is made.

Prior embarking on this project, I asked two young women living with endometriosis for their thoughts about the publication of a book focusing on endometriosis. In response to their comments detailing how the condition has impacted their physical, social and mental health, I felt there was a need to focus on inadequate primary care management, referral delays, red flag signs and symptoms and the role of specialist endometriosis centres. In the book, I have addressed the current barriers to effective care which include poor education about periods and what constitutes a normal menstrual cycle, stigma associated with discussing period problems and painful sex, and practitioners' lack of awareness of the symptoms and signs of endometriosis and the benefits of early intervention.

For a busy GP, there are simply not enough hours to read all the published guidance. I have, therefore, added in each chapter key points and useful references to direct further reading. These days, the primary care team includes other allied health care professionals such as advanced nurse practitioners, community nurses, physician associates, pharmacists and physiotherapists, all of whom will also find the book of value.

The report of the All-Party Parliamentary Group (APPG) on Endometriosis, published in 2020, found that there had been no significant improvement in care for women with endometriosis; in fact, further disruptions to care have resulted from pressure caused by the COVID-19 pandemic. I felt the need to set up the local Endometriosis Awareness North charity in 2020, addressing current challenges and priorities and to campaign for change. All the contributors of various chapters are working together to raise awareness of this condition, promote understanding through school and college education and raise funds for research.

Endometriosis in Primary Care: A Practical Guide is intended for general practitioners and other primary health care practitioners and medical students. It is all evidenced based. If you gain greater knowledge in management of patients with endometriosis and do a timely referral, the book will have served its purpose well.

Dr Anita Sharma

Acknowledgements

Every piece of writing takes time—time that could have been spent with my husband.

My heartfelt gratitude goes to my husband, Ravi, a consultant gastroenterologist, for his continued support and doing the household duties while I battled with my computer.

Above all, I would like to thank my son Neel, Founder and Director of Clinical Engineering Hub in Cambridge, who has written many medical books, for injecting energy and enthusiasm and motivating me at a time when a change in service delivery at the primary care level is very much needed.

General practice is facing many challenges and providing an ever-greater range of primary care services, but it is crucial that those services are provided in line with the latest evidenced-based guidelines.

This truly comprehensive book aims to equip GPs, GPs in training, medical students and allied health care professionals in primary care with the knowledge required to diagnosis endometriosis promptly and provide appropriate support to patients. Alongside guidelines for evidenced-based clinical practice, the book details other important issues such as women's health strategy, delayed diagnosis and comorbidities in women with endometriosis.

I am indebted to Dr Shalini Gadiyar, GP, who has a special interest in gynaecology, for her contribution towards complications of endometriosis focusing on fertility problems, one of the major issues. She describes how symptomatic endometriosis can have a significant and sometimes severe impact on the woman's quality of life including work productivity, relationships, sexual health, fitness and daily living.

Primary care is the first point of contact of a woman suffering with symptoms suggestive of endometriosis. I would like to thank both Courtney Ormrod and Lucy Bowker for making me focus on the chapters on symptoms of endometriosis and pharmacological management including non-drug management and timely referral as they both suffered a long delay in referral.

The surgical management of endometriosis is complex. I would like to thank Miss Gaity Ahmad, Clinical Director for Gynaecology, Clinical Lead for the NCA Endometriosis Centre and Honorary Senior Lecturer at Manchester University working in Royal Oldham Hospital and Rochdale Infirmary and her two registrars Dr Shatha Al-Attili and

Dr Jamel Tahar Aissa, focusing on what is endometriosis surgery, different types of surgery, who needs the surgery and what happens after the surgery including risks and complications. It is important for local GPs to know who to send the referral to, choosing the right consultant to avoid unnecessary delays.

Additional thanks go to Hannah Draper, speciality trainee and MD candidate and Professor Andrew Horne, Chair of the Academic Board at the RCOG, past Chair of the ESHRE Special Interest Group for Endometriosis and Endometrial Disorders, for contributing a chapter examining evidence supporting different surgical treatments including surgical management where fertility is a priority.

Menstrual health education programs in schools and colleges can help address a number of challenges including poor attendance, poor performance, lack of participation in school activities and friends making fun. I am particularly grateful to Margaret Heywood, the lead for school and college education for Endometriosis Awareness North who addresses the agenda of integrating menstrual learning within the curriculum in her contribution on "Education in Schools."

My special thanks to Catherine E.W. Pennington, Deborah P. Fischer, Professor Kay Marshall and Cohen J. Loveder for contributing towards the chapter on research, highlighting potential diagnostic and treatment options that may be on the horizon. At the time of writing this book, there is further research on the way which I have mentioned.

Finally, I thank Jo Koster for her continuing support and help with the preparation of manuscript.

Lead Author

Dr Anita Sharma, MBBS MD DRCOG MFFP, is a General Practitioner with a special interest in women's health in Oldham where she has been practising for over 30 years. She is also Educational Lead Northwest Family Doctors Association and a former Clinical Director for Vascular and Medicine Optimisation at Oldham Clinical Commissioning Group (CCG). She contributed towards setting up a community gynaecology clinic in Oldham to reduce pressure on the secondary care.

Dr Sharma served as a locality member in the West Pennine Local Medical Committee and was the Editor of the *LMC Newsletter.* She is Oldham's gynaecology triager and a GP appraiser for NHS England Northwest. She is Chair of the Women's Doctors Forum within the British International Doctors Association (BIDA), where her focus is on the Women's Health Strategy. The focus is not only on gynaecological and obstetrical issues but also the general wellbeing of women. She has given several talks on menopause and endometriosis to the BIDA division of Rochdale, Bolton, Blackburn and Wigan. She is an undergraduate trainer attached to the University of Manchester and is also involved with the University of Manchester and BRIT 2 project to help reduce antimicrobial prescribing. Previously she worked with Public Health England to address antimicrobial resistance (AMR). She has done various presentation for the Westminster forum on AMR strategy. She is the GP editor for the *British Journal of Medical Practitioners* and writes regularly in various GP magazines including *Pulse* on clinical and practice development issues and is a contributor to MIMS Learning CPD modules for health care professionals. She was a GP member of NICE Quality Standard Advisory Committee (QSAC) and Expert Advisors Panel for the NICE Centre for Guidelines for Endometriosis. At present, she is working with NICE to update menopause and breast cancer guidelines.

Dr Sharma has also produced previously recognized works in obstetrics and gynaecology winning in 2014 a first prize for *Gynaecology in Primary Care: A Practical Guide* (Radcliffe Publishing/CRC Press, 2013) at the British Medical Association Medical Book Awards. Her other books mainly aimed for primary care are *COPD in Primary Care* (Radcliffe Publishing/CRC Press, 2010), *Maximising Quality and Outcomes Framework Quality Points* (Radcliffe Publishing/CRC Press, 2011) and *Peripheral Vascular Disease in Primary Care* (Radcliffe Publishing/CRC Press, 2011).

Last year she developed the Endometriosis Awareness North Charity to help raise the awareness of endometriosis, the need for early diagnosis and management and to raise money for research. Andy Burnham, Mayor of Manchester, came to Oldham on 1st July 2023 to offer his support to her Charity. She is President of Rochdale Inner Wheel, and her chosen Charity is Endometriosis Awareness North.

Contributors

Gaity Ahmad
Department of Obstetrics and Gynaecology
Royal Oldham Hospital
Northern Care Alliance NHS Trust
Oldham, UK

Jamel Tahar Aissa
Department of Obstetrics and Gynaecology
Royal Oldham Hospital
Northern Care Alliance NHS Trust
Oldham, UK

Shatha Al-Attili
Department of Obstetrics and Gynaecology
Royal Oldham Hospital
Northern Care Alliance NHS Trust
Oldham, UK

Hannah Draper
Diana Princess of Wales Hospital
North Lincolnshire and Goole NHS Trust,
    Grimsby
Centre for Biomedicine
Hull York Medical School
University of Hull
Hull, UK

Deborah P. Fischer
Division of Pharmacy and Optometry
School of Health Sciences
Faculty of Biology
Medicine and Health
University of Manchester
Manchester, UK

Shalini Gadiyar
Ashworth Street Surgery
Rochdale, UK

Margaret Heywood
School and College Educator for
    Endometriosis Awareness North
Member of Patient Participation Group
Founder of Period Poverty Project Oldham
Cancer Aid Worker
Oldham, UK

Andrew Horne
Centre for Reproductive Health
Institute for Regeneration and Repair
University of Edinburgh
Edinburgh, UK

Cohen J. Loveder
Division of Pharmacy and Optometry
School of Health Sciences
Faculty of Biology
Medicine and Health
University of Manchester
Manchester, UK

Kay M. Marshall
Division of Pharmacy and Optometry
School of Health Sciences
Faculty of Biology
Medicine and Health
University of Manchester
Manchester, UK

Catherine E.W. Pennington
Division of Pharmacy and Optometry
School of Health Sciences
Faculty of Biology
Medicine and Health
University of Manchester
Manchester, UK

We also thank and acknowledge the following individuals for sharing their personal stories of living with endometriosis:

- Lucy Bowker and her father Tony Bowker
- Siobhan Kennett and her husband James Kennett
- Courtney Ormrod and her father Paul Ormrod

CHAPTER 1

Definition and Types of Endometriosis

....

Endometriosis is a disease characterized by the presence of tissue resembling endometrium (the lining of the uterus) outside the uterus (1). The tissue acts like regular uterine tissue does during the period. But this blood has nowhere to go. It causes a chronic inflammatory reaction that may result in irritation, severe pain, scarring, adhesions and fibrosis within the pelvis and other parts of the body. It is a benign, oestrogen dependent condition.

Globally, it affects 190 million women and those assigned female at birth, but a UK survey in 2017 reported that only 20% of the general public had ever heard of it.

Endometriosis has significant social, public health and economic implications. It can decrease quality of life due to severe pain, fatigue, depression, anxiety and infertility.

Addressing endometriosis will empower those affected by it by supporting their human right to the highest standard of sexual and reproductive health, quality of life and overall wellbeing.

Risk factors for endometriosis include (1,2):

- Early menarche
- Late menopause
- Delayed childbearing
- Nulliparity
- Late first sexual intercourse
- Smoking
- Low body mass index (BMI)

DOI: 10.1201/9781032684819-1

- Family history
- White ethnicity
- Vaginal outflow obstruction
- Autoimmune disease (an increased prevalence of autoimmune diseases has been noted in women with surgically confirmed endometriosis) (2)

At present, there is no known way to prevent endometriosis. Enhanced awareness, followed by early diagnosis and management, may slow or halt the natural progression of the disease and reduce the long-term burden of its symptoms, including possibly the risk of central nervous system pain sensitization but currently, there is no cure.

In the UK, work absenteeism and health care costs related to endometriosis cause economic losses of around £8.2 billion a year (direct treatment costs are comparable to those for type 2 diabetes and rheumatoid arthritis).

Earlier diagnosis and early treatment might reduce psychosocial and economic burdens.

According to retrospective population-linked data, delayed diagnosis was associated with a reduced chance of pregnancy by 33% in those who required assisted reproductive technology.

It is important to understand various types of endometriosis symptoms so that an early diagnosis is made.

Endometriosis lesions in the pelvis can be categorized as:

- Superficial peritoneal endometriosis (accounting for around 80% of endometriosis)
- Ovarian endometriosis (cysts or "endometrioma")
- Deep endometriosis (depth of penetration ≥5 mm)

Like eutopic endometrial tissue, the endometriosis lesions contain endometrial glands and stroma. The difference is that the endometriosis implants often contain fibrous tissue and blood. It is the breakdown of red blood cells which results in the formation of pigmented histocytes. The older the lesion, the more pigmented it is likely to be.

All forms of endometriosis can be found together, not solely as separate entities.

TYPES OF ENDOMETRIOSES

Several lesion types have been described based on where it is (3,4). The different types of disease may co-occur (i.e., a patient may have more than one type of disease present in the pelvis).

25–50%

OF WOMEN WITH ENDOMETRIOSIS HAVE OVARIAN ENDOMETRIOMAS

20%

OF WOMEN WITH ENDOMETRIOSIS HAVE A DEEP LESION

15%

OF WOMEN WITH DIGESTIVE ENDOMETRIOSIS HAVE LESIONS ON THE DIAPHRAGM

Superficial Peritoneal Lesion

This is the most common type. There are lesions on the peritoneum, a thin film that lines the pelvic cavity. While superficial peritoneal lesions classically contain endometrial glands and stroma, diagnostic challenges arise when there are alterations or absence of glandular or stromal components (5). The glandular components can be absent, sparse, or transformed by hormonal and metaplastic changes or cellular atypia. The stromal component can be obscured by infiltrates of foamy and pigmented histiocytes, fibrosis or other processes. Foci of endometriosis within the peritoneum are found in 15–50% of all women diagnosed with endometriosis. The best diagnostic method is to recognize them during laparoscopic surgery.

Inflammatory and reactive changes within or adjacent to foci of endometriosis can also cause confusion to the histological findings.

Histological diagnosis can also be hindered by a small biopsy sample.

Endometrioma (Ovarian Lesion)

These dark, fluid-filled cysts, also called chocolate cysts, form deep in the ovaries. They don't respond well to treatment and can damage healthy tissue. Both ovaries are involved in one-third of cases. Ovarian endometriosis occurs in 2–10% of women of reproductive age and 50% of patients treated for infertility.

In contrast with most haemorrhagic physiological ovarian cysts, endometriomas typically have fibrotic walls and surface adhesions; are filled with chocolate-coloured material; are surrounded by duplicated ovarian parenchyma (6); and are lined by endometrial epithelium, stroma and glands (7).

The endometrial epithelium and stroma lining the endometrioma can be lost over time and replaced by granulation tissue and dense fibrous tissue, which makes histological diagnosis difficult.

Varying in size from a few millimeters to several centimeters, these lesions are not intra-ovarian cysts. They are the result of intra-ovarian invagination of a lesion initially on the surface of the ovary which then progressively invaginates into the ovary. This makes the surgical treatment awkward as the endometrioma and the ovary are sometimes inseparable, which can lead to the damage of the ovary during removal of the cyst. Ovarian endometrioma can be diagnosed through imaging if the patient is referred early and the imaging is evaluated by an experienced imaging specialist.

Deep-Infiltrating Endometriosis

Deep-infiltrating endometriosis (DIE) is defined as a solid endometriosis mass situated more than 5 mm deep to the peritoneum (8). This type grows under the peritoneum and can involve organs near the uterus, such as bowels, bladder, ureter, rectovaginal septum, uterine ligaments and vagina (9). About 1% to 5% of women with endometriosis have this type.

These are hard, fibrous lesions in which hormone-dependent endometrial tissue is relatively little represented (15–20% of the volume of the endometriosis nodule). These lesions tend to infiltrate the surrounding organs and behave aggressively just like tumours, which makes the removal difficult.

Because of their fibrous composition and as they are not very hormone-dependent, the size of deep endometriosis nodules, little impacted by amenorrhoea, allows the disease to stabilize but rarely to disappear. This explains why they may be found in postmenopausal women despite amenorrhoea.

ANATOMIC SITES

In general, the most common sites of endometriosis, in decreasing order of frequency, are the ovaries, anterior and posterior cul-de-sac, posterior broad ligaments, uterosacral ligaments, uterus, fallopian tubes, sigmoid colon and appendix and round ligaments (10,11).

Occasionally, an endometrioma arises in the anterior abdominal wall, usually in the vicinity of a surgical incision (12), although these lesions can occur in women with no history of surgery or history of endometriosis.

Rare cases: Endometriosis has also been found outside the pelvis: Breast, pancreas, liver, gall bladder, kidney, urethra, vertebrae, bone, spleen, diaphragm, central nervous system, hymen (13) and lung (14). Other sites less commonly involved include vagina, cervix, rectovaginal septum, cecum, inguinal canal, ureters, urinary bladder and umbilicus.

Bowel Endometriosis

Endometriosis situated inside the bowel wall is termed "bowel endometriosis." It mostly affects the rectosigmoid area, but lesions can also be found in other parts of the gastrointestinal system, including the appendix.

Penetration of the endometriosis can vary within two forms:

- *Superficial*: Endometriosis is found on the surface of the bowel
- *Deep*: Endometriosis penetrates the bowel wall

In some cases, rectovaginal nodules can start as superficial endometriosis and progress to infiltrate the bowel wall. The usual treatment for bowel endometriosis is surgery. The surgical options vary depending on the severity of the endometriosis and the areas affected. Surgeries can be performed via a laparoscopy or via open surgery and may take several hours and more than one surgery depending on the extent of the endometriosis.

Endometriosis can affect patients in a variety of ways. In some, there are no symptoms; in others, their fertility is affected. With bowel endometriosis, the usual symptoms are pain on opening the bowels (dyschezia) and deep pelvic pain with sex (dyspareunia). Although bowel endometriosis can be associated with bleeding from the rectum during a period, this is perhaps more commonly caused by haemorrhoids (piles) and other bowel conditions.

Symptoms may vary with the menstrual cycle and are typically worse in the days before a period and during menstruation.

Bladder Endometriosis

Endometriosis involving the detrusor muscle and/or the bladder epithelium is termed "bladder endometriosis."

The bladder is the most common site affected in urinary tract endometriosis. There is controversy regarding the pathogenesis, clinical management (diagnosis and treatment), impact on fertility and risk of malignant transformation of bladder endometriosis (BE) (15).

Endometriosis affecting the bladder is rare and the exact cause is unknown. The penetration of the endometriosis can vary within two forms:

- *Superficial*: Endometriosis is found on the outer surface of the bladder
- *Deeper*: Endometriosis is found on the inside of the bladder lining or wall, which can cause a nodule, and can also affect the ureter

Symptoms of bladder endometriosis can vary with the menstrual cycle, tending to be worst in the days before and during a period. Most common symptoms are urgency, occasional haematuria and pain when bladder is full. Cystoscopy and laparoscopy are the diagnostic tests. If deep endometriosis is suspected, a CT and/or MRI scan is done to confirm the diagnosis.

BE is a challenging condition, and the common coexistence of other types of endometrioses means that clinical management of BE should involve collaboration between gynaecologists and urologists.

The surgical options vary depending on the severity and the area of the bladder affected.

Excision of the Lesion

Clinical management can be conservative, using hormonal therapies, or surgical. When conservative treatment is preferred, oestrogen-progestogen combinations and progestogens should be chosen because of their favourable profile that allows long-term therapy. Surgery should guarantee complete removal of the bladder nodule to minimize recurrence, so transurethral surgery alone should be avoided in favour of segmental bladder resection. There is not a strong rationale for hypothesizing a detrimental impact of BE per se on fertility. Furthermore, current evidence does not support the removal of bladder endometriotic lesions because of the potential risk of malignant transformation since this phenomenon is exceedingly rare (15).

Extra-Abdominal Endometriosis

Extra-abdominal (replacing the older term "extra-pelvic") endometriosis is used to describe any endometriosis lesions found outside of the abdomen, for example, thoracic endometriosis (16), hepatic, brain or ocular.

Thoracic Endometriosis

The presence of endometrial tissue in the thoracic cavity is called thoracic endometriosis (TE). Thoracic endometriosis is rare, and it can be hard to identify. It can take up to 4 years to identify the condition. There can be active endometrial tissue in the tracheobronchial tree, lung parenchyma and lung pleura. Many women who have thoracic endometriosis also have the more common pelvic form of endometriosis. Between 50–84% of women with thoracic endometriosis also have pelvic endometriosis. While thoracic endometriosis can develop spontaneously, it typically affects people with a history of severe pelvic endometriosis.

Pulmonary endometriosis has four main clinical conditions: namely catamenial pneumothorax, catamenial haemothorax, catamenial haemoptysis and endometrial nodules in the lung.

Brain Endometriosis

Endometriosis of the brain is a rare condition that can occur without cyclical symptoms related to menstruation. Cerebral endometriosis is the growth of endometrial tissue in the brain. Cerebral endometriosis is extremely rare, with only three cases reported to date in scientific literature. One involved a reported case of cerebellar endometriosis, or endometrial cells found in the back part of the brain known as the cerebellum.

Hepatic Endometriosis

Hepatic endometriosis is one of the rarest disorders characterized by the presence of ectopic endometrium in the liver. To our knowledge, only 21 cases of hepatic endometrioma have been described in medical literature (17).

Ocular Endometriosis

Ocular endometriosis is a rare, underdiagnosed subtype, with no established pathogenesis, diagnostic criteria or means of treatment.

Endometrial tissue is also hypothesized to travel lymphatically or hematogeneously to reach extra-pelvic organs like the eye.

A thorough review of the available literature has shown that the anatomic location of ocular endometriosis renders it even harder to diagnose, preventing physicians from obtaining a biopsy for a definitive diagnosis or excising it to provide treatment. Moreover, the eye was shown to be responsive to hormonal changes occurring in the menstrual cycle, which cease to occur in physiologic states like pregnancy or while on exogenous ovarian suppression regimens.

> The case report by Barat and Kwedar (1988) described a 17-year-old girl who experienced intermittent bleeding from her right eye during her menstrual cycle. These bleeding episodes occurred about 10 times per day, each lasting 2 to 3 minutes. They began with retro-orbital pain and pressure that ceased once her eye started bleeding. She also experienced right-sided headaches that were relieved by acetaminophen and codeine (18).

Abdominal Wall Endometriosis

Abdominal wall endometriosis is a rare clinical condition with unclear pathophysiology. It occurs frequently after gynaecologic or obstetric surgery. This pathology will be encountered more frequently considering the increasing rate of caesarean section (19).

The most common symptoms are abdominal pain with abdominal wall mass during menstruation. Ultrasonography, computed tomography (CT scan) and MRI are useful for diagnosis.

Abdominal wall endometriosis management is surgical excision. Excision goals are to remove the mass and to confirm histological diagnosis of parietal endometriosis.

ENDOMETRIOSIS VS. ADENOMYOSIS

Adenomyosis and endometriosis are both disorders of the endometrial tissue that lines the inside of the uterus. But they develop differently and have some different symptoms. In adenomyosis, endometriotic deposits form in the myometrium (the muscle of the uterus).

Adenomyosis is not a sub-phenotype of endometriosis (20), although it is characterized by endometrial tissue surrounded by smooth muscle cells within the myometrium (21). In these patients, there will be symptoms of painful periods and heavy menstrual and/or abnormal uterine bleeding.

These misplaced cells follow the menstrual cycle and bleeding monthly. The uterus wall thickens and may cause pain and heavy bleeding. It usually affects older people and is associated with infertility.

Risk Factors for Adenomyosis

- Higher body mass index (BMI)
- Use of oral contraceptives
- Increased exposure to oestrogen such as starting periods at an early age or having multiple pregnancies

- Use of oral contraceptives
- History of uterine surgeries such as caesarean section (C-section), fibroid removal or dilatation and curettage (D&C)
- Use of tamoxifen

Causes of Adenomyosis

The cause of adenomyosis is not known. Menopause usually relieves adenomyosis symptoms. Some people with endometriosis may still have symptoms after menopause, though this isn't very common.

There have been many theories including:

- *Invasive tissue growth*: Some experts believe that endometrial cells from the lining of the uterus invade the muscle that forms the uterine walls. Uterine incisions made during an operation such as a caesarean section (C-section) might promote the direct invasion of the endometrial cells into the wall of the uterus
- *Developmental origins*: Other experts suspect that endometrial tissue is deposited in the uterine muscle when the uterus is first formed in the fetus
- *Uterine inflammation related to childbirth*: Another theory suggests a link between adenomyosis and childbirth. Inflammation of the uterine lining during the postpartum period might cause a break in the normal boundary of cells that line the uterus
- *Stem cell origins*: A recent theory proposes that bone marrow stem cells might invade the uterine muscle, causing adenomyosis

Regardless of how adenomyosis develops, its growth depends on the body's circulating oestrogen.

Symptoms

Adenomyosis is more common in multiparous women than nulliparous women. The average age of diagnosis is between 40 and 50 years of age. However, this disease can occur in young women as well as after menopause. Both adenomyosis and endometriosis can be painful over time. Both are progressive disorders, but they're treatable and not life-threatening.

Symptoms of adenomyosis include heavy menstrual bleeding, prolonged periods, chronic pelvic pain, infertility and an enlarged uterus. Pain can range from mild to severe. Approximately 60% of women with adenomyosis experience abnormal uterine bleeding and 25% experience dysmenorrhea (pelvic pain during menstruation).

Adenomyosis is also associated with other uterine disorders. More than 80% of women with adenomyosis have another abnormal condition in the uterus; 50% of patients have associated fibroids, approximately 11% have endometriosis most commonly in the ovaries and 7% have endometrial polyps. The symptoms of these associated conditions often make it difficult to diagnose adenomyosis.

Diagnosis

Early diagnosis and treatment can lead to a better outcome for pain and symptom relief. The range of diagnosis of adenomyosis varies between 5% and 70% of patients. Pelvic ultrasound scan or pelvic MRI may suggest this condition but cannot positively diagnose it. The only way to conclusively diagnose the condition is through surgery to examine the uterus.

Treatment

The right treatment depends on a person's symptoms and fertility goals. The only definitive treatment for adenomyosis is total hysterectomy. Gonadotropin-releasing hormone (GnRH) agonists can help by inducing amenorrhoea, but recurrence of symptoms occur within 6 months of stopping GnRH treatment.

Oral contraceptives, nonsteroidal anti-inflammatory drugs (NSAIDs) and danazol can help symptom control in those who wish to preserve future fertility. One may need fertility treatments to get pregnant such as intrauterine insemination (IUI) and in vitro fertilization (IVF).

The good news is that there are many ongoing studies on adenomyosis and endometriosis.

ENDOMETRIOSIS VS. ENDOMETRITIS

Endometritis and endometriosis are two different conditions. Both conditions refer to the endometrium.

Endometritis occurs in the uterus, while endometriosis occurs outside the uterus.

The suffix of each word can help distinguish the two conditions.

Endometritis is irritation or inflammation of the endometrium. It is usually due to infection, or a pelvic procedure done through the cervix. Common *symptoms of endometritis* include:

- Abdominal pain or swelling
- Pelvic pain

- Painful or uncomfortable bowel movements
- Constipation
- Abnormal vaginal bleeding
- Unusual or heavy vaginal discharge
- Fever
- Feeling unwell
- Trouble conceiving/Miscarriage

Causes of Endometritis

The causes of endometritis are somewhat less complex than those of endometriosis. In most cases, the condition results from some sort of infection in the uterus including:

- Sexually transmitted infection (STI) such as chlamydia or gonorrhoea
- A secondary tuberculosis infection in the genital tract that results from tuberculosis lung infection
- After an event such as miscarriage, prolonged labour, caesarean section (C-section), endometrial biopsy or dilation and curettage (D&C)
- Following intra uterine contraception device (IUCD) insertion

Diagnosis

Diagnostic testing should be done to confirm a diagnosis of endometritis or to rule out other conditions, including endometriosis:

- Tender abdominal and pelvic examination
- FBC (Full Blood Count), ESR (Erythrocyte Sedimentation rate)
- Vaginal and cervical swabs, and if caused by an STI, sexual partners must be notified
- Endometrial biopsy to exclude endometrial cancer

Treatment

Treating endometritis is often less complex than treating endometriosis. It involves treating the infection with appropriate antibiotics orally or intravenously depending on the severity of infection. Treating sexually transmitted infections, making sure sexual partners are treated for STIs and following safe-sex practice reduces the risk of endometritis.

KEY POINT SUMMARY

- Endometriosis lesions in the pelvis can be categorized as superficial peritoneal endometriosis, ovarian endometriosis and deep endometriosis.
- The most common sites of endometriosis, in decreasing order of frequency, are the ovaries, anterior and posterior cul-de-sac, posterior broad ligaments, uterosacral ligaments, uterus, fallopian tubes, sigmoid colon and appendix and round ligaments.
- Rarely reported sites include brain, eyes, breast, pancreas, liver, gall bladder, kidney, urethra, vertebrae, bone and spleen.
- Deep-infiltrating endometriosis (DIE): Deep-infiltrating endometriosis is the most severe type of endometriosis, causing lesions to spread and grow deep into the pelvic region.
- Both adenomyosis and endometriosis may make it harder to get pregnant.
- Endometritis and endometriosis are separate conditions that may present similar symptoms. Endometritis can be caused by an STI, tuberculosis, or vaginal infection. Often, endometritis is preceded by an event such as a C-section or an overly long labour. Untreated endometritis can cause symptoms such as pelvic pain, constipation and infertility.

REFERENCES

1. Coleman L, Overton C. GPs have a key role in early diagnosis of endometriosis. *Practitioner* 2015; 259(1780):13. (Abstract)
2. BMJ. *Endometriosis*. BMJ Best Practice. 2019. www.bestpractice.bmk.com
3. World Health Organization (WHO). *International classification of diseases, 11th revision (ICD-11)*. Geneva: WHO, 2018.
4. Johnson NP, Hummelshoj L, Adamson GD, et al. World endometriosis society consensus on the classification of endometriosis. *Hum Reprod* 2017;32(2):315–24.
5. Clement PB. The pathophysiology of endometriosis: A survey of the many faces of a common disease emphasizing diagnostic pitfalls and unusual and newly appreciated aspects. *Adv Anat Pathol* 2007;14:241.
6. Brosens IA, Puttemans PJ, Deprest J. The endoscopic localization of endometrial implants in the ovarian chocolate cyst. *Fertil Steril* 1994;61:1034.
7. Muzil L, Bianchi A, Bellati F, et al. Histological analysis of endometriomas: What the surgeon needs to know. *Fertil Steril* 2007;87:362.
8. De Cicco C, Corona R, Schonman R, et al. Bowel resection for deep endometriosis: A systematic review. *BJOG* 2011;118:285.
9. Woodward PJ, Sohaey R, Mezzetti TP, Jr. Endometriosis: Radiologic-pathologic correlation. *Radiographics* 2001;21:193.
10. Gustofson RL, Kim N, Liu S, et al. Endometriosis and the appendix: A case series and comprehensive review of the literature. *Fertile Steril* 2006;86:298.
11. Jenkins S, Olive DL, Haney AF. Endometriosis: Pathogenetic implications of the anatomic distribution. *Obstet Gynecol* 1986;67:335.

12. Dwivedi AJ, Agarwal SN, Silva YJ. Abdominal wall endometriomas. *Dig Dis Sci* 2002;47:456.
13. Canlorbe G, Laas E, Cortez A, et al. Spontaneous hymeneal endometriosis: A rare cause of dyspareunia. *BMJ Case Rep* 2014;2014.
14. Redwine DB. Diaphragmatic endometriosis: Diagnosis, surgical management, and long-term results of treatment. *Fertil Steril* 2002;77:288.
15. Leone Roberti Maggiore U, Ferrero S, Candiani M, et al. Bladder endometriosis: A systematic review of pathogenesis, diagnosis, treatment, impact on fertility, and risk of malignant transformation. doi:10.1016/j.eururo.2016.12.015
16. Andres MP, Arcoverde FVL, Souza CCC, et al. Extrapelvic endometriosis: A systematic review. *J Minim Invasive Gynecol* 2020;27:373–89. doi:10.1016/j.jmig.2019.10.004 pmid:31618674 [CrossRef] [PubMed] [Google Scholar]
17. Liu K, Zhang W, Liu S, et al. Hepatic endometriosis: A rare case and review of the literature. 2015. doi:10.1186/s40001-015-0137-1 pmid:25886632 pmcid:PMC4389341
18. Barat M, Kwedar SA. Ocular vicarious menstruation. *J Pediatr Ophthalmol Strabismus* 1988;25:254–5. [PubMed] [Google Scholar]
19. Ferjaoui MA, Arfaoui R, Khedhri S, et al. Abdominal wall endometriosis: A challenging iatrogenic disease. *Int J Surg Case Rep* 2021 Nov;88:106507. doi:10.1016/j.ijscr.2021.106507 (accessed 14 Oct 2021).
20. Halvorson LM. New perspectives on adenomyosis. *Semin Reprod Med* 2020;38:87–8. doi:10.1055/s-0040-1721376 pmid:33232984 [CrossRef] [PubMed] [Google Scholar]
21. Bulun SE, Yildiz S, Adli M, et al. Adenomyosis pathogenesis: Insights from next-generation sequencing. *Hum Reprod Update* 2021;27:1086–97. doi:10.1093/humupd/dmab017 pmid:34131719 [CrossRef] [PubMed] [Google Scholar]

FURTHER READING

Adenomyosis-NHS. www.nhs.uk/conditions/Adenomyosis
BMJ. *Endometriosis.* BMJ Best Practice. 2019. www.bestpractice.bmk.com
NHS Inform Website. *Adenomyosis.* www.nhsinform.scot/healthy-living/womens-health/girls-and-young-women-puberty-to-around-25/periods-and-menstrual-health/adenomyosis (accessed 12 Oct 2023).
World Health Organization (WHO). *International classification of diseases, 11th revision (ICD-11).* Geneva: WHO, 2018.

CHAPTER 2

Staging and Classification

································

Endometriosis is a challenging disease to classify, as it is known to have different phenotypes and presentations (both with regards to the type of lesions and their location) and various symptoms without a clear link to presentation. Moreover, the natural progression of the disease is unknown.

There is a perceived need for a validated classification or descriptive system for endometriosis that could support further progress in defining subgroups and, more importantly, guiding the therapeutic options for women with pain and/or infertility. Such a system would certainly also progress endometriosis research by unifying patient subgroups and facilitating the development of prognostic and predictive tools.

Classification and staging systems are widely used in medicine and have been shown to be valuable in guiding clinical management. Examples include the American Joint Committee on Cancer (AJCC) tumour-node-metastasis (TNM) staging systems for cancer and the Gleason score for prostate cancer. But in the field of endometriosis, several classification, staging and reporting systems have been developed.

Twenty-two endometriosis classification, staging and reporting systems were published between 1973 and 2021 (1), each developed for specific, and different, purposes. There still is no international agreement on how to describe the disease or how to classify it, and most classification/staging systems show little or no correlation with patient outcomes.

A few studies confirm the value of the ENZIAN system for surgical description of deep endometriosis. With regard to infertility, the Endometriosis Fertility Index has been confirmed to be valid for its intended purpose.

DOI: 10.1201/9781032684819-2

The three most commonly used systems are:

- Revised American Society for Reproductive Medicine (rASRM) Classification (stages I–IV; where stage I is equivalent to "minimal" disease and stage IV to "severe" disease)
- ENZIAN (and newer #ENZIAN) Classification
- Endometriosis Fertility Index (EFI) (2–5)

THE REVISED AMERICAN SOCIETY FOR REPRODUCTIVE MEDICINE (rASRM) CLASSIFICATION

The classification developed by the American Society of Reproductive Medicine (ASRM), based on the results of laparoscopy or laparotomy, is the most common system used in clinical practice. The most important goal of classifying and determining the severity of endometriosis is to propose an effective treatment plan for it (6).

The American Society of Reproductive Medicine distinguishes four stages of endometriosis, where stage I and II are mild types, and stages III and IV are advanced disease (7,8).

Staging depends on location, extent and depth of the adhesions:

- *Stage I (1–5 points)*: This is a minimal form of the disease. There may be a few small adhesions or tiny lesions. These may appear on one ovary or the tissue lining the pelvis or abdomen. There's little to no scar tissue
- *Stage II—(6–15 points)*: This is a mild form, with more lesions, occurring at a deeper level. It can affect both ovaries, and there is scar tissue but usually no inflammation
- *Stage III—(16–40 points)*: This refers to a moderate level of the disease. It may present small cysts on one or both ovaries and thick adhesions. Areas like the peritoneum and cul de sac will also be affected
- *Stage IV—(> 40 points_)*: This is considered severe endometriosis, with deep lesions and thick adhesions. There are also large cysts on one or both ovaries and their tubes. This may require more than one kind of treatment and multiple surgeries

The rASRM system (scored at surgery based on the extent of visualized superficial peritoneal lesions, endometriomas and adhesions) has been shown to have poor correlation with pain (9), fertility outcomes and prognosis.

> A large impediment is the lack of routine, harmonized documentation of the characteristics of endometriosis and its absence from international classification of diseases coding (10).

ENZIAN SYSTEM

The ENZIAN classification was introduced in Austria in 2005 (3). The ENZIAN score, like the rASRM classification, is determined by the extent of endometriosis during surgery. When the ENZIAN classification was first developed, its purpose was not to compete with the rASRM classification but to supplement it with respect to the description of DIE. However, according to Haas et al. (11), there was unintended partial overlapping with the rASRM score.

Therefore, two revisions of the ENZIAN classification system were carried out in 2010 and 2011 to correct the overlap between the rASRM and ENZIAN systems and to make it easier to use (12,13). The revised ENZIAN classification was simplified by dividing retroperitoneal structures into three compartments. The posterior part of the uterus was divided into compartment A consisting of the rectovaginal septum and vagina, compartment B consisting of the uterosacral ligament and pelvic walls, and compartment C consisting of the sigmoid colon and rectum. The severity of the lesion is set to invasiveness <1 cm for grade 1, invasiveness 1 to 3 cm for grade 2 and invasiveness >3 cm for grade 3.

The prefix "E" indicates the presence of a tumour of endometriosis. The number that follows the prefix indicates the size of the lesion, and after the number, the lowercase English letter indicates the affected compartment. Two lowercase English letters mean bilateral disease. The invasion of endometriosis to other organs in the pelvic cavity and to distant organs is expressed as follows: "FA" is defined as adenomyosis, "FB" as involvement of the bladder, "FU" as intrinsic ureter involvement, "FO" as involvement of other locations and "FI" as intestinal involvement. This revision is helpful for physicians to better understand and readily use the ENZIAN classification.

One of the advantages of the ENZIAN classification is that it provides detailed descriptions of the retroperitoneal structures. The compartment can be divided into three sections, and the severity of each compartment as well as that of the distant lesions, such as diaphragmatic and ureteral invasions, can be described. Second, the ENZIAN classification can be determined by imaging modalities and used for surgical planning. A study has reported that magnetic resonance imaging (MRI) predicts the extent of disease before surgery using ENZIAN score and enables preoperative surgical planning. The accuracy of the ENZIAN scores detected by preoperative MRI was 95% with a low false-negative rate of 4% (14). Third, disease localization and extent, as described by the revised ENZIAN score, are associated and correlate with the presence and severity of different symptoms (15).

However, there are several drawbacks. First, the ENZIAN classification has a poor level of international acceptance. It is currently not widely used but mainly used in German-speaking countries. Second, patients may not readily understand the ENZIAN classification because of the complexity of the stage and insufficient knowledge of the pelvic anatomy. If there is a 2-cm unilateral infiltration of endometriosis, the ENZIAN classification expresses it as "E2b." This terminology does not accurately convey the severity of the disease to the patient. Third, the ENZIAN score will be inaccurate if the surgical dissection of the deep invasive lesions is incompletely performed or if image study alone is performed without surgery. Fourth, even if the ENZIAN classification is predicted by imaging modalities, there is insufficient research regarding the usefulness of the classification determined by imaging.

The ENZIAN system additionally includes deep endometriosis. This has been shown to have poor correlation with symptoms and infertility (16,18).

To date, there is no gold standard for the classification of endometriosis. Only expert consensus regarding the current classification systems exists. The World Endometriosis Society (WES) released a consensus statement on the classification of endometriosis in 2017. International experts from 29 organizations systematically evaluated the classification of endometriosis and reached this consensus (17).

The WES suggested that the following recommendations should be considered in critical situations. All women undergoing surgery must complete rASRM classification to obtain the maximum information until better classification is available, and women with DIE must additionally complete ENZIAN classification. EFI must be additionally completed in women who need to consider fertility in future (17).

The recommendation is that until better classification systems have been developed, surgeons should use a toolbox for surgical classification of endometriosis (that includes the rASRM system and, where appropriate, the ENZIAN and EFI staging systems) to maximize the information available to women following their surgery (17).

Further study is needed to clarify whether the preoperative ENZIAN score can be used for evaluating the surgical feasibility or complete resectability.

The ENZIAN scale in deep-infiltrating endometriosis is a descriptive scale, considering both the existence of the lesion and the depth of the invasion. In the ENZIAN classification, the location of foci was assigned to separate anatomical compartments (19).

Coding of the Recorded Findings

P = Peritoneum (diameter of that circle in which the areas of all visible foci can be summarized fictitiously $=\Sigma$).
- P1 = <3 cm
- P2 = 3–7 cm
- P3 = >7 cm (Detection by surgery)

O = Ovary (sums of diameters of all endometriosis cysts; each side assessed separately: left/right).
- O1 = <3 cm
- O2 = 3–7 cm
- O3 = >7 cm

A *Detection by US/MRI/Surgery*

T   = Adhesions and tubo-ovarian findings (adhesions of adnexa to pelvic wall, uterus and bowel, tubal patency= +/–; each side assessed separately; li/re)

T1 = Adhesions of ovary to pelvic wall

T2 = Adhesions of ovary, pelvic wall and uterus

T3 = Adhesions of ovary, pelvic wall, uterus and intestine

B Detection by US/Surgery

A/B/C = Deep endometriosis
    A = Retrocervical area, septum rectovaginale, vagina
    B = Parametrium, ligamentum sacrouterinum
    C = Rectosigmoid
- Assessment of size, that is, diameter in each case

C Detection by TVS/MRI/Surgery

F = FA = Adenomyosis
    FI = Other intestinal lesions >16 cm from anus
    FU = Ureter(left/right), obstruction
 F(. . .) = Defined other localizations
- Detection by TVS/MRI/surgery

The #ENZIAN classification can be applied intraoperatively, by sonography or with MRI and is annotated with the small letters: (s) = Surgery, (u) = Ultrasound, (m) = MRI.

Each of these diagnostic methods has specific strengths and weaknesses. For example, peritoneal lesions cannot be visualized and classified sonographically, or occasionally a bowel lesion cannot be visualized and classified sufficiently well by diagnostic laparoscopy alone. A combination of the findings of the different methods is possible and also useful.

If anatomic structures cannot be assessed (e.g., due to extensive adhesions), the affected compartment is coded with an (x).

Only those compartments showing pathology are coded to make the extent of the disease with the affected organs easier and faster to understand.

ENDOMETRIOSIS FERTILITY INDEX (EFI)

This is a well-validated clinical tool that predicts pregnancy rates after surgical staging of endometriosis, with ongoing evaluation to determine the predictive importance of the individual parameters included in the scoring algorithm as well as the effect of completeness of surgical treatment on pregnancy prediction (20).

The purpose of the development of the EFI system is to predict the pregnancy rate in patients with surgically documented endometriosis who have not attempted to become pregnant with in vitro fertilization (IVF).

The EFI system reflects historical factors such as age, duration of infertility and previous pregnancies. For pregnancy, proper functioning of the fallopian tube, fimbria and ovary is required. The functional score indicates whether the embryo is well implanted into the uterus, whether the uterus can provide an early environment for the embryo, or whether the fallopian tubes can pick up the ovum well.

Functional scores are determined by the surgeon and range from 0 to 4 points as follows; absent or nonfunctional as 0, severe dysfunction as 1, moderate dysfunction as 2, mild dysfunction as 3 and normal as 4. Not only the least functional score but also other surgical factors such as rASRM total score and endometriosis lesion score of rASRM are included. Finally, the EFI score is calculated by summing the historical and surgical scores and ranges from 0 to 10 points, with 10 indicating the best prognosis and 0 the worst prognosis.

The EFI system has a clear advantage on predicting pregnancy outcome. The EFI score reflects the pregnancy rate better than the rASRM classification does. According to Zeng et al. (21), the pregnancy rate was 53.6%, 36.0%, 51.7% and 41.7% in rASRM stages I, II, III and IV, respectively, with no statistically significant difference ($p = 0.246$). However, the pregnancy rate according to the EFI score was observed to be statistically significant at 8.3% in the group with an EFI score of 0 to 3, 41.2% for a score of 4 to 7 and 60.9% for a score of 8 to 10 ($p < 0.001$) (21). Similarly, the EFI score is a more reliable system to predict IVF outcomes in endometriosis patients than the rASRM classification. Wang et al. (22) reported that the IVF outcomes were higher in patients with an EFI score of 6 or higher than in those with a score of 5 or less.

However, the EFI system has the following disadvantages. First, the EFI score does not correlate with pain. Second, as the least function score is judged subjectively, the total score can vary by surgeon. To date, there is no study on the assessments of interobserver reliability and intra-observer reproducibility in the EFI system. Third, the EFI score is more complicated to use than the rASRM classification and ENZIAN score since it requires the calculation and addition of the scores of various categories.

Women with a high EFI score have excellent fertility prognosis and may be advised to try to become pregnant with timed intercourse compared to women with a low score, for whom a prompt referral to assisted reproductive technology (ART) seems more reasonable (20).

The location and impact of lesions on the ability of the adnexa to function seems crucial for the fertility prognosis and should be investigated further (20).

The EFI system was developed to make a prognostic statement about the probability of pregnancy in endometriosis and infertility.

This multifactorial statistical model takes into account not only endometriosis but also other factors that limit fertility, such as the age of the patient, previous pregnancies, the duration of infertility, the state of the tubo-ovarian entity and, finally, the rASRM stage.

The points calculated in this process give an estimation of the prognosis for a spontaneous pregnancy. However, of the maximum 10 points to be scored, only 2 points are given specifically for endometriosis staging. Thus, the EFI cannot be considered primarily as a specific endometriosis classification.

The ENZIAN classification, which has been updated and modified recently in the form of the so-called #ENZIAN classification, has proved to be the most suitable tool for staging DE and now also includes peritoneal or ovarian diseases as well as adhesions. In the ideal scenario, a classification for endometriosis can be used with both diagnostic and surgical methods. The present work discusses the pros and cons of scores for endometriosis and highlights the need for using one universal classification system (23).

KEY POINT SUMMARY

- Correct staging of endometriosis is of great importance for both diagnosis and therapy.
- The application of the ENZIAN classification shows high clinical applicability and accuracy, especially for DE, and can also be used noninvasively with TVS and MRI.
- A universally useable system such as the updated #ENZIAN system may allow for complete classification of endometriosis using non-invasive and invasive techniques.
- The ENZIAN classification, which has been updated and modified recently in the form of the so-called #ENZIAN classification, has proved to be the most suitable tool for staging DE and now also includes peritoneal or ovarian diseases as well as adhesions (23).

REFERENCES

1. Vermeulen N, Abrao MS, Einarsson JI, et al. International working group of AAGL, ESGE, ESHRE and WES. Endometriosis classification, staging and reporting systems: A review on the road to a universally accepted endometriosis classification. *Hum Reprod Open* 2021;2021:hoab025. doi:10.1093/hropen/hoab025 pmid:34693032 [CrossRef] [PubMed] [Google Scholar]
2. Revised American Society for Reproductive Medicine classification of endometriosis: 1996. *Fertil Steril* 1997;67:817–21. doi:10.1016/S0015-0282(97)81391-X pmid:9130884 [CrossRef] [PubMed] [Web of Science] [Google Scholar]
3. Tuttlies F, Keckstein J, Ulrich U, et al. [ENZIAN-score, a classification of deep infiltrating endometriosis]. *Zentralbl Gynakol* 2005;127:275–81. doi:10.1055/s-2005-836904 pmid:16195969 [CrossRef] [PubMed] [Google Scholar]
4. Adamson GD, Pasta DJ. Endometriosis fertility index: The new, validated endometriosis staging system. *Fertil Steril* 2010;94:1609–15. doi:10.1016/j.fertnstert.2009.09.035 pmid:19931076 [CrossRef] [PubMed] [Google Scholar]
5. Keckstein J, Saridogan E, Ulrich UA, et al. The #ENZIAN classification: A comprehensive non-invasive and surgical description system for endometriosis. *Acta Obstet Gynecol Scand* 2021;100:1165–75. doi:10.1111/aogs.14099 pmid:33483970 [CrossRef] [PubMed] [Google Scholar]
6. Szamatowicz M. Endometriosis—Still an enigmatic disease. What are the causes, how to diagnose it and how to treat successfully? *Gynecol Endocrinol* 2008;24:535–6. doi:10.1080/09513590802296062 [PubMed] [CrossRef] [Google Scholar]
7. Damario MA, Rock JA. Classification of endometriosis. *Semin Reprod Endocrinol* 1997;15:235–44. doi:10.1055/s-2008-1068753. [PubMed] [CrossRef] [Google Scholar]
8. Gilmour JA, Huntington A, Wilson HV. The impact of endometriosis on work and social participation. *Int J Nurs Pract* 2008;14:443–8. doi:10.1111/j.1440-172X.2008.00718.x [PubMed] [CrossRef] [Google Scholar]

9. Schliep KC, Mumford SL, Peterson CM, et al. Pain typology and incident endometriosis. *Hum Reprod* 2015;30:2427–38. doi:10.1093/humrep/dev147 pmid:26269529 [CrossRef] [PubMed] [Google Scholar]

10. Whitaker LHR, Byrne D, Hummelshoj L, et al. Proposal for a new ICD-11 coding classification system for endometriosis. *Eur J Obstet Gynecol Reprod Biol* 2019;241:134–5. doi:10.1016/j.ejogrb.2019.08.015 pmid:31477250 [CrossRef] [PubMed] [Google Scholar]

11. Haas D, Chvatal R, Habelsberger A, et al. Comparison of revised American Fertility Society and ENZIAN staging: A critical evaluation of classifications of endometriosis on the basis of our patient population. *Fertil Steril* 2011;95:1574–8. [PubMed] [Google Scholar]

12. Stiftung Endometriose Forschung 6th Conference of the Stiftung Endometriose Forschung (Foundation for Endometriosis Research); 2010 Feb 19–21; Weissensee, Austria. Stiftung Endometriose Forschung. [Google Scholar]

13. Stiftung Endometriose Forschung the revised ENZIAN classification. Consensus meeting, 7th Conference of the Stiftung Endometriose Forschung (Foundation for Endometriosis Research); 2011 Feb 25–27; Weissensee, Austria. [Google Scholar]

14. Di Paola V, Manfredi R, Castelli F, et al. Detection and localization of deep endometriosis by means of MRI and correlation with the ENZIAN score. *Eur J Radiol* 2015;84:568–74. [PubMed] [Google Scholar]

15. Montanari E, Dauser B, Keckstein J, et al. Association between disease extent and pain symptoms in patients with deep infiltrating endometriosis. *Reprod Biomed Online* 2019;39:845–51. [PubMed] [Google Scholar]

16. Haas D, Shebl O, Shamiyeh A, et al. The rASRM score and the ENZIAN classification for endometriosis: Their strengths and weaknesses. *Acta Obstet Gynecol Scand* 2013;92:3–7. doi:10.1111/aogs.12026 pmid:23061819 [CrossRef] [PubMed] [Google Scholar]

17. Johnson NP, Hummelshoj L, Adamson GD, et al. World Endometriosis Society Sao Paulo Consortium. World Endometriosis Society consensus on the classification of endometriosis. *Hum Reprod* 2017;32:315–24. doi:10.1093/humrep/dew293 pmid:27920089 [CrossRef] [PubMed] [Google Scholar]

18. Andres MP, Borrelli GM, Abrão MS. Endometriosis classification according to pain symptoms: Can the ASRM classification be improved? *Best Pract Res Clin Obstet Gynaecol* 2018;51:111–18. doi:10.1016/j.bpobgyn.2018.06.003 pmid:30029959 [CrossRef] [PubMed] [Google Scholar]

19. Tuttlies F, Keckstein J, Ulrich U, et al. ENZIAN-score, a classification of deep infiltrating endometriosis. *Zentralbl Gynakol* 2005;127:275–81. [PubMed] [Google Scholar]

20. Maheux-Lacroix S, Nesbitt-Hawes E, Deans R, et al. Endometriosis fertility index predicts live births following surgical resection of moderate and severe endometriosis. *Hum Reprod* 2017;32:2243–9. doi:10.1093/humrep/dex291 pmid:29040471 [CrossRef] [PubMed] [Google Scholar]

21. Zeng C, Xu JN, Zhou Y, et al. Reproductive performance after surgery for endometriosis: Predictive value of the revised American Fertility Society classification and the endometriosis fertility index. *Gynecol Obstet Invest* 2014;77:180–5. [PubMed] [Google Scholar]

22. Wang W, Li R, Fang T, et al. Endometriosis fertility index score maybe more accurate for predicting the outcomes of in vitro fertilisation than r-AFS classification in women with endometriosis. *Reprod Biol Endocrinol* 2013;11:112. [PMC free article] [PubMed] [Google Scholar]

23. Keckstein J. Gernot Hudelist Classification of deep endometriosis (DE) including bowel endometriosis: From r-ASRM to #ENZIAN-classification. doi:10.1016/j.bpobgyn.2020.11.004. Epub 2020 Dec 11.

FURTHER READING

Brosens IA. Classification of endometriosis revisited. *Lancet* 1993;341:630. doi:10.1016/0140-6736(93)90389-X. [PubMed] [CrossRef] [Google Scholar]

Damario MA, Rock JA. Classification of endometriosis. *Semin Reprod Endocrinol* 1997;15:235–44. doi:10.1055/s-2008-1068753. [PubMed] [CrossRef] [Google Scholar]

CHAPTER 3

Prevalence

....

Endometriosis affects roughly 10% (190 million) of reproductive age women and girls globally (1), but a survey done in UK in 2017 reported that only 20% of the general public had ever heard of it (2).

Endometriosis is also reported in women after menopause, but where that occurs, it is thought to have developed prior to menopause without earlier detection (3,4).

Determining the prevalence of endometriosis in the general population is challenging because some women are asymptomatic, those with symptoms have varied and nonspecific presentations and definitive diagnosis requires surgery (5).

Prevalence Estimates

- A 2017 cross-sectional survey of nearly 60,000 women in the US estimated the prevalence of confirmed endometriosis at 6.1%, with symptom burden greatest in those aged 18–29 (6)
- A 2021 population-based survey in Australia reported that 6.3% of women aged 40–44 have clinically confirmed endometriosis (7)
- Population prevalence is estimated at 10%, based on prevalence estimates of pelvic pain and infertility in the general population (8)
- In four studies of mainly asymptomatic women undergoing tubal ligation, the prevalence of endometriosis ranged from 1–7% (9)

DOI: 10.1201/9781032684819-3

Prevalence in Certain Patient Groups

- In 2% to 11% of women, endometriosis is an incidental finding during surgery for other indications (10)
- 7% to 43.3% among women undergoing tubal sterilization (11)
- Up to 50% of women presenting with infertility and 24–40% of those with chronic pelvic pain have endometriosis (1,12,13)
- In a retrospective cohort study of over 9,500 women undergoing laparoscopic or abdominal hysterectomy for benign indications, 15% of women were diagnosed with endometriosis (14)
- Endometriosis has been reported in up to 40% of adolescents with genital tract anomalies (15)

The Ghiasi meta-analysis reported (16) prevalence estimates for endometriosis widely varied from 0.2% to 71.4% depending on the population sampled. The prevalence reported in general population studies ranged from 0.7% to 8.6%, whereas that reported in single clinic- or hospital-based studies ranged from 0.2% to 71.4%.

When defined by indications for diagnosis, endometriosis prevalence ranged from 15.4% to 71.4% among women with chronic pelvic pain, 9.0% to 68.0% among women presenting with infertility and 3.7% to 43.3% among women undergoing tubal sterilization. A meta-regression was conducted with year as the predictor of prevalence. No trend across time was observed among "general population in country/region" studies ($\beta = 0.04$, $p = 0.12$) or among "single hospital or clinic" studies ($\beta = -0.02$, $p = 0.34$); however, a decrease over time was observed among general population studies abstracted from health systems or insurance systems ($\beta = -0.10$, $p = 0.005$).

Population sampling and study design matters. Heterogeneity of inclusion and diagnostic criteria and selection bias overwhelmingly account for variability in endometriosis prevalence. It is difficult to conclude if the lack of observed change in frequency and distribution of endometriosis over the past 30 years is valid.

ESHRE guideline endometriosis offers best practice advice on the care of women with endometriosis, including recommendations on the diagnostic approach and treatments for endometriosis for both relief of painful symptoms and for infertility due to endometriosis (17).

This hypothesis is supported by a recent report from a large US health system's electronic medical records database that observed a decline from 2006 through 2015 in incidence rates for endometriosis (from 30.2 per 10,000 person-years in 2006 to 17.4 per 10,000 person-years in 2015) but an increase in documentation of chronic pelvic pain diagnoses (from 3.0% to 5.6%) (18).

BARRIERS TO CARE IN THE UK

If endometriosis is estimated to affect 1.5 million women in the UK, a prevalence comparable to the number of women with diabetes (19), why is there such a poor knowledge and under recognition of this condition? Why do so many women feel unsupported?

A new report by the all-party parliamentary group on women's health shows:

- 42% of women said that they were not treated with dignity and respect
- 62% of women were not satisfied with the information that they received about treatment options for fibroids and endometriosis
- Nearly 50% of women with endometriosis and fibroids were not told about the short-term or long-term complications from their treatment

The All-Party Parliamentary Group on Women's Health has found that women are not being treated appropriately when it comes to their gynae-cological health.

This report reveals some of the barriers that women faced in getting a diagnosis and treatment, and the complete lack of control and choice they were offered over their own care.

The report also sets out the key issues that are important to patients and crucial for their care:

- Symptoms and concerns should be taken seriously and not dismissed and/or ignored
- Timely referral to appropriate specialist care is needed
- Information about all possible treatment options and their side effects and complications should be offered

This report also highlighted:

- 40% of women with endometriosis needed 10 GP appointments or more before being referred
- 39% of women sought a second opinion
- 67% of women said they got most of their information from the internet

APPG recommends:

- *Information resources*: Women need to be offered written information with a full range of details about the condition and what their options are. These leaflets should be endorsed by the relevant clinical bodies and patient groups, and the same generic, pre-approved leaflets should be made available at all centres, trusts and gynaecology clinics. GPs, secondary care clinicians and nurses should provide or signpost women to high-quality information and resources about endometriosis, its impact and treatment options
- *Endorsed best practice pathway*: This would mean that women would be streamlined more quickly into the right care, saving costs from unplanned admissions and ensuring women get access to all treatments. This should be agreed by the relevant Royal Colleges and patient groups
- *Education to include menstrual health at secondary schools along with wider awarenes*: Far too often, women put up with symptoms and incredible pain because they are not aware of what is "normal" and they feel stigmatized by talking about "women's problems"
- *Multidisciplinary teams and clinicians working together*: To ensure access to all treatments for women, teams should work together, and the best practice pathway should be followed in this regard
- *NICE Guidance, where it exists, should be followed*: These should not be implemented variably across the country as is currently the situation

Main barriers include:

- Stigma associated with discussing period problems and painful sex, especially among Black and minority ethnic (BAME) women
- Lack of awareness of symptoms and not seeking early help from a GP
- Poor education at schools and colleges. Patients and practitioners lack of awareness of the symptoms and signs of endometriosis and the benefits of early intervention
- Delayed investigations

The All Party Parliamentary Group (APPG) on Endometriosis' 2020 report, *Endometriosis in the UK: Time for Change* (19), found that there had been no significant improvement in care for women with endometriosis—in fact, further disruptions to care have resulted from pressures caused by the COVID-19 pandemic (15,20).

In 2017, NICE published NICE Guideline 73, *Endometriosis: Diagnosis and Management* (21) to raise awareness of the symptoms of endometriosis and optimize its management in health care settings, but no real difference has been observed in early diagnosis or early management.

Factors Associated with Increased Risk

- Nulliparity (22)
- Prolonged exposure to endogenous oestrogen—early menarche (before the age of 11 to 13 years (23)
- Late menopause (24)
- Shorter menstrual cycle (defined as < 27 days) (22)
- Heavy menstrual bleed (22)
- Lower BMI (22). A low body mass index has long been considered a key risk factor for development of endometriosis. Normal BMI 18.5 to 24.9. If the BMI is less than 18.5 it is low
- Height greater than 68 inches (23)
- Obstruction to menstrual blood flow (24)
- Exposure to severe physical and/or sexual abuse in childhood or adolescence (25)
- High consumption of trans unsaturated fat (26)

Factors Associated with Decreased Risk

- Multiple births (27)
- Late menarche (after the age of 14 years (23)
- Race may also be a risk factor, as the prevalence has been reported being higher in White and Asian women compared with Black and Hispanic women (27)
- Ovarian endometriomas were less common in those women who used oral contraceptive pills compared with women who had not (28)

KEY POINT SUMMARY

- The exact prevalence of endometriosis is unknown given diagnostic delays and barriers.
- A recent meta-analysis identified 69 studies describing the prevalence and/or incidence of endometriosis, among which 26 studies were general population samples, 17 were from regional/national hospitals or insurance claims systems, and the remaining 43 studies were conducted in single clinic or hospital settings (16).
- The Ghiasi meta-analysis reported a decrease in recorded prevalence across the past 30 years, which could be due to more rapid and empiric treatment (16).

- While the prevalence varies with the population being studied, approximately 10% of reproductive age women globally have endometriosis.
- Determining the prevalence of endometriosis in the general population is challenging because some women are asymptomatic, those with symptoms have varied and nonspecific presentations and definitive diagnosis requires surgery.

REFERENCES

1. World Health Organization (WHO). *International classification of diseases, 11th Revision (ICD-11)*. Geneva: WHO, 2018.
2. Horne AW, Saunders PTK, Abokhrais IM, et al. Endometriosis priority setting partnership steering group (appendix). Top ten endometriosis priorities in the UK and Ireland. *Lancet* 2017;389:2191–2. doi:10.1016/S0140-6736(17)31344-2 pmid:28528751.
3. Marsh EE, Laufer MR. Endometriosis in premenarcheal girls who do not have an associated obstructive anomaly. *Fertil Steril* 2005;83:758–60. doi:10.1016/j.fertnstert.2004.08.025
4. Oxholm D, Knudsen UB, Kryger-Baggesen N, et al. Postmenopausal endometriosis. *Acta Obstet Gynecol Scand* 2007;86:1158–64. doi:10.1080/00016340701619407
5. Hickey M, Ballard K, Farquhar C. Endometriosis. *BMJ* 2014;348:g 1752.
6. Endometriosis. *BMJ* 2022;379. doi:10.1136/bmj-2021-068950 (Published 28 Nov 2022) Cite this as: *BMJ* 2022;379:e068950.
7. Fuldeore MJ, Soliman AM. Prevalence and symptomatic burden of diagnosed endometriosis in the United States: National estimates from a cross-sectional survey of 59 411 women. *Gynecol Obstet Invest* 2017;82:453–61. doi:10.1159/000452660 pmid:27820938
8. Rowlands IJ, Abbott JA, Montgomery GW, et al. Prevalence and incidence of endometriosis in Australian women: A data linkage cohort study. *BJOG* 2021;128:657–65. doi:10.1111/1471-0528.16447 pmid:32757329 [CrossRef] [PubMed] [Google Scholar]
9. Sangi-Haghpeykar H, et al. Epidemiology of endometriosis among parous women. *Obstet Gynecol* 1995;85:983.
10. Ye L, Whitaker LHR, Mawson RL, et al. Endometriosis. *BMJ* 2022 Nov 28;379:e068950. doi:10.1136/bmj-2021-068950.
11. Horne AW, Missmer SA. Pathophysiology, diagnosis, and management of endometriosis. *BMJ* 2022;379. doi:10.1136/bmj-2022-070750 (Published 14 Nov 2022) Cite this as: *BMJ* 2022;379:e070750.
12. Shafrir AL, Farland LV, Shah DK. Risk for and consequences of endometriosis: A critical epidemiologic review. *Best Pract Res Clin Obstet Gynaecol* 2018;51:1–15. doi:10.1016/j.bpobgyn.2018.06.001 [CrossRef] [PubMed] [Google Scholar]
13. Eskenazi B, Warner ML. Epidemiology of endometriosis. *Obstet Gynecol Clin North Am* 1997;24:235–58. doi:10.1016/S0889-8545(05)70302-8 pmid:9163765 [CrossRef] [PubMed] [Web of Science] [Google Scholar]
14. Mowers EL, Lim CS, Skinner B, et al. Prevalence of endometriosis during abdominal or laparoscopic hystrectomy for chronic pelvic pain. *Obstet Gynecol* 2016;127:1045.

15. Dovey S, Sanfilippo J. Endometriosis and the adolescent. *Clin Obstet Gynecol* 2010;53:420.
16. Ghiasi M, Kulkarni MT, Missmer SA. Is endometriosis more common and more severe than it was 30 years ago? *J Minim Invasive Gynecol* 2020;27:452–61. doi:10.1016/j.jmig.2019.11.018 pmid:31816389 [CrossRef] [PubMed] [Google Scholar]
17. Becker CM, Bokor A, Heikinheimo O, et al. ESHRE Endometriosis Guideline Group ESHRE guideline: Endometriosis. *Hum Reprod Open* 2022;2022:hoac009. doi:10.1093/hropen/hoac009 pmid:35350465 [CrossRef] [PubMed] [Google Scholar]
18. Christ JP, Yu O, Schulze-Rath R, et al. Incidence, prevalence, and trends in endometriosis diagnosis: A United States population-based study from 2006 to 2015. *Am J Obstet Gynecol* 2021;225:500.e1–9. doi:10.1016/j. ajog.2021.06.067 pmid:34147493
19. All Party Parliamentary Group on Endometriosis, Endometriosis UK. *Endometriosis in the UK: Time for change.* London: Endometriosis UK, 2020. www.endometriosis-uk.org/sites/default/files/files/Endometriosis%20 APPG%20Report%20Oct%202020.pdf (accessed 11 Feb 2023).
20. Spencer J, Mezquita G, Shakir F. The ongoing impact of the COVID-19 pandemic on endometriosis patients: A survey of 1,089 UK patients. *Facts Views Vis Obgyn* 2022;14(3):257–64.
21. NICE. *Endometriosis: Diagnosis and management.* NICE Guideline 73. NICE, 2017. www.nice.org.uk/ng73 (accessed 11 Feb 2023).
22. Ballard KD, Seaman HE, de Vries CS, et al. Can symptomatology help in the diagnosis of endometriosis? Findings from a national case-control study—Part 1. *BJOG* 2008;115:1382.
23. Treloar SA, Bell TA, Nagle CM, et al. Early menstrual characteristics associated with subsequent diagnosis of endometriosis. *Am J Obstet Gynecol* 2010;202:534.e1.
24. Giudice LC. Clinical practice: Endometriosis. *N Engl J Med* 2010;363:2389.
25. Harris HR, Wieser F, Vitonis AF, et al. Early life abuse and risk of endometriosis. *Hum Reprod* 2018;33:1657.
26. Missmer SA, Chavarro JE, Malspeis S, et al. A prospective study of dietary fat consumption and endometriosis risk. *Hum Reprod* 2010;25:1528.
27. Missmer SA, Hankinson SE, Spiegelman D, et al. Incidence of laparoscopically confirmed endometriosis by demographic, anthropometric and lifestyle factors. *Am J Epidemiol* 2004;160:784.
28. Kavoussi SK, Odenwald KC, As-Sanie S, et al. Incidence of ovarian endometrioma among women with peritoneal endometriosis with and without a history of hormonal contraceptive use. *Eur J Obstet Gynecol Reprod Biol* 2017;215:220.

FURTHER READING

All Party Parliamentary Group on Endometriosis, Endometriosis UK. *Endometriosis in the UK: Time for change.* London: Endometriosis UK, 2020. www. endometriosis-uk.org/sites/default/files/files/Endometriosis%20APPG%20 Report%20Oct%202020.pdf (accessed 11 Feb 2023).
Endometriosis UK website. *Endometriosis facts and figures.* www.endometriosis-uk. org/endometriosis-facts-and-figures (accessed 11 Feb 2023).
NICE. Endometriosis: *Diagnosis and management.* NICE Guideline 73. NICE. 2017. www.nice.org.uk/ng73 (accessed 11 Feb 2023).

CHAPTER 4

Causes and Risk Factors

....

Endometriosis is a complex disease that affects some women globally, from the onset of their first period (menarche) through menopause regardless of ethnic origin or social status.

No one currently knows the exact cause of endometriosis. Genetics, lifestyle and environment are believed to play a major role. There are also certain risk factors that may increase the likelihood of developing endometriosis, although they tend to be non-modifiable (such as age or family history). It is not clear what can be done to reduce one's personal risk other than to exercise regularly and generally maintain optimal health. Doing so may reduce high oestrogen levels that contribute to the severity and frequency of symptoms (1).

Several hypotheses have been proposed to explain the origins of endometriosis:

- **Retrograde menstruation:** According to the most common theory of ectopic endometrial cells (Sampson's theory of retrograde menstruation), endometrial cells flow backwards through the fallopian tubes into peritoneal cavity during menses, at the time that blood is flowing out of the body through the cervix and vagina (2).

    Other potential sources of ectopic endometrial cells include mesothelium, stem cells, Müllerian rests (3), bone marrow stem cells (3), lymphatic or vascular dissemination (4) and coelomic metaplasia (5).

    Evidence supporting retrograde menstruation comes from the observation that the incidence of endometriosis is increased in girls with genital tract obstructions that prevent drainage of menses through the vagina and, therefore, increase tubal reflux (6).

DOI: 10.1201/9781032684819-4

However, while up to 90% of women have retrograde menstruation (7), most women do not develop endometriosis, which suggests that additional factors are involved.

- *Induction theory*: This theory proposes that certain hormones or immune factors may inadvertently transform certain cells of the peritoneum (the lining of the peritoneal cavity) into endometrial cells.

  The hypothesis of induction theory is supported by animal research in which uterine tissues grafted onto the peritoneum of baboons induced endometriosis. Later evaluation of the tissues found that they were biologically distinct from the endometrial lesions that naturally occur with endometriosis.

  The theory may better explain why prepubescent girls get endometriosis, as well as why certain cases of endometriosis affect distant organs such as the brain, lungs or skin (8). It is still unclear which factor or combination of factors (such as hormones, autoimmune disease, toxins, among others) may act as the "trigger" for endometrial induction.

- *Cellular metaplasia*: A process by which cells in the pelvic and abdominal area change into endometrial type cells of the germinal epithelium. This theory could explain how endometriotic cells appear spontaneously in the body and how they appear in areas such as the lung and skin. It could also explain why endometriosis occurs in some women after hysterectomy and in men taking hormone treatment (9).

- *Immune dysfunction*: Many women with endometriosis appear to have reduced immunity to other conditions. It is not known whether this contributes to endometriosis or whether it is because of endometriosis (9).

- *Stem cells*: Stem cells can give rise to the disease, which then spreads through the body via blood and lymphatic vessels.

- *Embryonic cell theory*: This suggests that the oestrogen may inadvertently transform undifferentiated embryonic cells into endometrial cells during puberty (10). This means that residual embryonic cells in the developing female reproductive tract may persist after birth and be induced into endometriosis under the influence of oestrogen. This may explain why some younger girls get endometriosis given that puberty will usually begin in girls between the ages of 8 and 14.

  This theory does not explain the cases where endometriosis develops outside of the female reproductive tract. Some scientists believe that this occurs when dislodged endometrial cells are transported by the lymphatic system to distant parts of the body, the same way as lymphoma and metastatic cancers (11).

- *Genetic predisposition*: Most scientists agree that genetics play a large part in the development of endometriosis. Statistics alone provide evidence to support this. Women's risk of endometriosis is between 7 and 10 times greater if she has a first-degree relative (such as mother or sister) with endometriosis. Beyond the inheritance of genes, genetics may also contribute indirectly by influencing hormone production.

   Even having a second- or third-degree relative with endometriosis can increase the risk. There are currently no genetic tests available that can reliably identify or predict the risk of endometriosis (12,13).

   It is believed that endometriosis is caused not by one but multiple genetic mutations (14). They may be somatic mutations (which occur after conception and cannot be inherited), germline mutations (which are passed to offspring), or a combination of the two.

   Scientists have identified several genetic mutations closely linked to endometriosis, including:

   - 7p15.2, which influences uterine development
   - GREB1/FN1, which helps regulate oestrogen production
   - MUC16, responsible for forming protective mucus layers in the uterus
   - CDKN2BAS, which regulates tumour suppressor genes believed to be linked to endometriosis
   - VEZT, which aids in the creation of tumour suppressor genes
   - WNT4, which is vital to the development of the female reproductive tract

   Beyond the inheritance of genes, genetics may also contribute indirectly by influencing hormone production. Endometriosis commonly occurs in the presence of persistently elevated oestrogen levels (15).

- *Environmental factors*: This theory suggests that certain environmental toxins can affect the body immune system and reproductive system and cause endometriosis. Animal studies have shown the development of endometriosis in animals following exposure to high levels of dioxin (9).

ROLE OF OESTROGEN RECEPTOR β IN ENDOMETRIOSIS

Endometriosis is known to be dependent on oestrogen, which facilitates the inflammation, growth and pain associated with the disease.

Endometriosis commonly occurs in the presence of persistently elevated oestrogen levels (15).

The biologically active oestrogen, oestradiol, aggravates the pathological processes (e.g., inflammation and growth) and the symptoms (e.g., pain) associated with endometriosis.

Abundant quantities of oestradiol are available for endometriotic tissue via several mechanisms including local aromatase expression. The question remains, then, what mediates oestradiol action. Because oestrogen receptor (ER)β levels in endometriosis are >100 times higher than those in endometrial tissue, this review focuses on this nuclear receptor (16).

Deficient methylation of the ERβ promoter results in pathological overexpression of ERβ in endometriotic stromal cells. High levels of ERβ suppress ERα expression. A severely high ERβ-to-ERα ratio in endometriotic stromal cells is associated with suppressed progesterone receptor and increased cyclo-oxygenase-2 levels contributing to progesterone resistance and inflammation. ERβ-selective oestradiol antagonists may serve as novel therapeutics of endometriosis in the future (16).

Aromatase excess syndrome (AEX) is an extreme example in which high oestrogen output is linked to a specific genetic mutation.

However, the relationship between oestrogen and endometriosis is complex since the absence of oestrogen does not always preclude the presence of endometriosis.

Once endometriosis is established, the process appears to cause symptoms through inflammatory changes. Endometriosis-related pelvic pain is associated with increased production of inflammatory and pain mediators as well as neurologic dysfunction related to implants (17). An increase of nerve fibres and imbalance of sympathetic and sensory nerve fibres (18) have been demonstrated in women with endometriosis-related pain. Oestrogen acting as a neuromodulator that selectively repulses the sympathetic axons while preserving sensory innervation is the proposed mechanism for pain symptoms. The mechanism for subfertility appears to involve anatomic distortion from pelvic adhesions and endometriomas and/or production of substances (e.g., cytokines, growth factors, prostanoids) that are hostile to ovulation, fertilization and implantation.

OTHER RISK FACTORS

Beyond a familial risk, there are several other characteristics typically seen in women with endometriosis. However, it is not surprising when a person with endometriosis does have one or a few of these risk factors present.

Age

Endometriosis affects women of reproductive age, usually between 15 and 49 (19). While it can sometimes develop before a girl's first period, endometriosis usually occurs several years after the onset of menstruation.

Most cases are identified between the ages of 25 and 35 (20), the time in life when many women are trying to get pregnant. In many such women, infertility may be the first overt sign of endometriosis (or the one that compels them to seek medical attention).

Estimates suggest that between 20% and 50% of women being treated for infertility have endometriosis, according to a 2010 review of studies in the *Journal of Assisted Reproduction and Genetics.*

Body Mass Index (BMI)

A low body mass index (BMI) has long been considered a key risk factor for the development of endometriosis. (This is contrary to many health disorders in which a high BMI contributes to disease risk.)

According to a 2017 review (21) involving 11 clinical trials, the risk of endometriosis was 31% less in women with a BMI over 40 (defined as obese) than women of normal weight (BMI of 18.5 to 24.9). Even compared to overweight women, women with obesity had a lower overall risk of endometriosis.

Menstrual Cycle

There are certain menstrual cycle characteristics that are commonly experienced in women with endometriosis (22):

- Starting period before the age of 12
- Having short menstrual cycles, generally less than 27 days
- Experiencing heavy periods lasting longer than 7 days
- Going through menopause at an older age

The longer one is exposed to oestrogen (either by starting menstruation early or ending late), the greater is the risk for endometriosis.

The same applies to the severity of menstrual symptoms, which commonly occurs with high oestrogen levels.

Sexual Activity during Menstruation

Sexual activity during menstruation can be a predisposing risk factor for endometriosis. Proper health education for women of reproductive age can promote their health and prevents endometriosis. Sexual activity during menstruation may increase the risk of retrograde menstrual bleeding, thereby increase the probability of seeding endometrial tissue in places other than the endometrial cavity (23).

Uterine Abnormalities

Uterine abnormalities may increase the risk of endometriosis by facilitating retrograde menstruation. These include conditions that alter the position of the uterus or obstruct the menstrual flow. Examples include:

- Uterine fibroids
- Uterine polyps
- Retrograde uterus (also known as a tilted uterus) in which the uterus curves in a backward position at the cervix rather than forward.
- Congenital uterus malformations, including cryptomenorrhea (in which menstruation occurs but cannot be seen due to a congenital obstruction)
- Asynchronous vaginal contractions, in which the vagina contracts abnormally and/or excessively during menstruation

Pregnancy Characteristics

Women who have never been pregnant are at greater risk of endometriosis (24). It is unclear whether this is solely a risk factor for endometriosis or if it is the consequence of infertility that affects nearly one of every two women with the disease.

On the flip side, pregnancy and breastfeeding are associated with a reduced risk of endometriosis (25). They do so by prolonging the absence of menstrual periods (postpartum amenorrhea), thereby reducing the level of oestrogen and other hormones associated with endometriosis symptoms.

Contrary to popular belief, pregnancy does not "cure" endometriosis. It may provide temporary relief (particularly if combined with breastfeeding), but it doesn't eradicate the underlying endometrial overgrowth (25).

In some cases, endometriosis may go away completely with the onset of menopause (unless one is taking oestrogen).

Abdominal Surgery

Abdominal surgeries like a caesarean section or hysterectomy can sometimes displace endometrial tissue. Any remaining tissues not destroyed by the immune system may implant themselves outside of the uterus, leading to endometriosis.

A 2013 analysis (26) from Sweden concluded that women who had a caesarean section with their first child were 80% more likely to be later diagnosed with endometriosis than those who delivered vaginally.

No risk was seen after two or more caesarean sections.

Lifestyle

Lifestyle plays less of a role in the development of endometriosis than one might imagine. This makes mitigating the risk even more challenging given that there are few modifiable factors one can change.

One can reduce the chances of developing endometriosis by lowering the levels of oestrogen in the body. This is especially true if one has known risk factors for endometriosis, including family history, polymenorrhagia or cryptomenorrhea.

The following steps can help lower and normalize oestrogen levels:

- Exercising regularly, ideally more than 4 hours per week
- Reducing alcohol intake to no more than one drink per day
- Cutting back on caffeine, ideally to no more than one caffeinated drink per day

Regular exercise is thought to promote reduced menstrual flow, ovarian stimulation and oestrogen effects (27).

Cardiovascular activity helps endometriosis patients maintain good energy levels. Exercise is one of the most effective strategies for increasing serotonin levels; physical activity and deep breathing exercises can increase the rate of burning serotonin neurons in the brain, which can stimulate the production of mood-enhancing substances. Aerobic exercise, such as walking and swimming, can have a more significant effect on serotonin levels, strengthening the muscles of the whole body and improving overall circulation (28).

Diet

Diet plays a very important role in preventing the development of endometriosis. The consumption of green vegetables and fresh fruits is considered to be the most beneficial (29). They contain antioxidants, which play an important role in the proper functioning of the immune system and the removal of free radicals. It is worth noting that the fibre contained in vegetables interacts in the control of the intestinal bacterial flora and affects hormonal balance.

Red meat exerts an antagonistic effect on the development of endometriosis compared to vegetables and fruits. It is characterized by a high content of dioxins, hormones and fat, increasing the concentration of oestrogens (29).

In the latest research by the team of Yamamoto et al., an attempt was made to determine whether higher consumption of red meat, poultry, fish and seafood is associated with the risk of laparoscopically confirmed endometriosis (30). The study group consisted of 81,908 women, and the observations covered the years from 1991 to 2013. Diet was assessed using a properly prepared nutrition questionnaire administered every 4 years. It was shown that respondents who reported eating > 2 servings/day of red meat had a 56% higher risk of endometriosis compared to those consuming ≤ 1 serving/week. Women who were classified in the category that consumed the most red meat were more likely to have endometriosis. No association with poultry, fish, shellfish and egg consumption and the risk of endometriosis was demonstrated (30).

A very important factor in the prevention of primary endometriosis is the maintenance of an appropriate lifestyle, in which a significant part should be occupied by rest, movement and physical activity (30).

Somatic Mutation

The association of endometriosis with cancer, which appears as a result of genetic mutations, has contributed to the search for pathogenetic mutations occurring in cells during the development of the disease. The concept of this research is based on the hypothesis that at least some of the changes arise because of somatic mutations that are absent in the germline and occur during the development of an individual organism. The occurrence of de novo mutations in both the endometrial cyst epithelial and peritoneal foci as well as in DIE foci is described. The most frequently noted genes are: ARID1A, KRAS, PIK3CA and PPP2R1A (31,32).

KEY POINT SUMMARY

- The exact cause of endometriosis is unclear. There are a few theories of how endometriosis starts but no confirmed cause.
- Elevated oestrogen levels appear to be a factor in the development of endometriosis.
- Genetics, lifestyle and environment also play a role.
- Having a first-degree relative with endometriosis increases the risk for developing endometriosis by 7–10 times.

REFERENCES

1. Bonocher C, Montenegro M, Rosa e Silva J, et al. Endometriosis and physical exercises: A systematic review. *Reprod Biol Endocrinol* 2014;12(1):4. doi:10.1186/1477-7827-12-4
2. Sampson JA. Peritoneal endometriosis due to the menstrual dissemination of endometrial tissue into the peritoneal cavity. *Am J Obstet Gynecol* 1927;14:422–69.
3. Burney RO, Giudice LC. Pathogenesis and pathophysiology of endometriosis. *Fertil Steril* 2012;98:511.
4. Javert CT. The spread of benign and malignant endometrium in the lymphatic system with a note on coexisting vascular involvement. *Am J Obstet Gynecol* 1952;64:780.
5. Gruenwald P. Origin of endometriosis from the mesenchyme of the celomic walls. *Am J Obstet Gynecol* 1942;44:470.
6. Dovey S, Sanfilippo J. Endometriosis, and the adolescent. *Clin Obstet Gynecol* 2010;53:420.
7. Halme J, Hammond MG, Hulka JF, et al. Retrograde menstruation in healthy women and in patients with endometriosis. *Obstet Gynecol* 1984;64:151.
8. Samani E, Mamillapalli R, Li F, et al. Micrometastasis of endometriosis to distant organs in a murine model. *Oncotarget* 2017;10(23). doi:10.18632/oncotarget.16889
9. Endometriosis UK. *Understanding endometriosis-information pack.* Endometriosis UK. 2012. www.endometriosis-uk.org.
10. Makiyan Z. Endometriosis origin from primordial germ cells. *Organogenesis* 2017;13(3):95–102. doi:10.1080/15476278.2017.1323162
11. Jerman L, Hey-Cunningham A. The role of the lymphatic system in endometriosis: A comprehensive review of the literature. *Biol Reprod* 2015;92(3). doi:10.1095/biolreprod.114.124313
12. Hickey M, Ballard K, Farquhar C. Endometriosis. *BMJ* 348.
13. BMJ. Endometriosis BMJ Best Practice. 2019. www.bestpractice.bmj.com
14. Dun E, Taylor R, Wieser F. Advances in the genetics of endometriosis. *Genome Med* 2010;2(10):75. doi:10.1186/gm196
15. Dyson M, Bulun S. Cutting SRC-1 down to size in endometriosis. *Nat Med* 2012;18(7):1016–18. doi:10.1038/nm.2855
16. Bulum SE, Monsavais D, Pavone ME, et al. Role of estrogen receptor–B in endometriosis. *Semin Reprod Med* 2012 Jan;30(1):39–45. doi:10.1055/s-0031-1299596. Epub 2012 Jan 23.
17. Anaf V, Simon P, El Nakadi I, et al. Relationship between endometriotic foci and nerves in rectovaginal endometriotic nodules. *Hum Reprod* 2000;15:1744.
18. Arnold J, Barcena de Arellano ML, Ruster C, et al. Imbalance between sympathetic and sensory innervation in peritoneal endometriosis. *Brain Behav Immun* 2012;26:132.
19. von Theobald P, Cottenet J, Iacobelli S, et al. Epidemiology of endometriosis in France: A large, nation-wide study based on hospital discharge data. *Biomed Res Int* 2016;2016:1–6. doi:10.1155/2016/3260952
20. Endometriosis: MedlinePlus Medical Encyclopedia. Medlineplus.gov.
21. Liu Y, Zhang W. Association between body mass index and endometriosis risk: A meta-analysis. *Oncotarget* 2017;8:46928–36. doi:10.18632/oncotarget.14916
22. Wei M, Cheng Y, Bu H, et al. Length of menstrual cycle and risk of endometriosis. *Medicine (Baltimore)* 2016;95(9):e2922. doi:10.1097/md.0000000000002922
23. Mollazadeh S, Najmabadi KM, Mirghafourvand M, et al. Sexual activity during menstruation as a risk factor for endometriosis: A systematic review

and meta-analysis. *Int J Fertil Steril* 2023 Jan–Mar;17(1):1–6. Published online 2022 Dec 25. doi:10.22074/IJFS.2022.541102.1207

24. Ashrafi M, Sadatmahalleh SJ, Akhoond MR, et al. Evaluation of risk factors associated with endometriosis in infertile women. *Int J Fertil Steril* 2016;10(1):11–21.

25. Leeners B, Damaso F, Ochsenbein-Kölble N, et al. The effect of pregnancy on endometriosis—facts or fiction? *Hum Reprod Update* 2018;24(3):290–9. doi:10.1093/humupd/dmy004

26. Andolf E, Thorsell M, Kallen K. Caesarean section and risk for endometriosis: A prospective cohort study of Swedish registries. doi:10.1111/1471-0528.12236

27. Warren MP, Perlroth NE. The effects of intense exercise on the female reproductive system. *J Endocrinol* 2001;170:3–11. doi:10.1677/joe.0.1700003. [PubMed]

28. Carpenter SE, Tjaden B, Rock JA, Kimball A. The effect of regular exercise on women receiving danazol for treatment of endometriosis. *Int J Gynaecol Obstet* 1995;49:299–304. doi:10.1016/0020-7292(95)02359-K. [PubMed]

29. Parazzini F, Chiaffarino F, Surace M, et al. Selected food intake and risk of endometriosis. *Hum Reprod* 2004;19:1755–9. doi:10.1093/humrep/deh395. [PubMed]

30. Yamamoto A, Harris HR, Vitonis AF, et al. A prospective cohort study of meat and fish consumption and endometriosis risk. *Am J Obstet Gynecol* 2018;219:178. e1–178.e10. doi:10.1016/j.ajog.2018.05.034. [PMC free article] [PubMed]

31. Zondervan KT, Becker CM, Missmer SA. Endometriosis. *N Engl J Med* 2020;382:1244–56. doi:10.1056/NEJMra1810764. [PubMed]

32. Redwine D. Regarding should genetics now be considered the pre-eminent etiologic factor in endometriosis? *J Minim Invasive Gynecol* 2020;27:1426–7. doi:10.1016/j.jmig.2020.03.015. [PubMed] [CrossRef]

FURTHER READING

BMJ. 2019. Endometriosis BMJ Best Practice. www.bestpractice.bmj.com
Endometriosis UK. 2012. www.endometriosis-uk.org
WHO World Health Organisation 11th revision (ICD-11). Geneva: WHO, 2018.

CHAPTER 5

Symptoms

....

Endometriosis, also called "endo," is a chronic disease. The most common symptom is pain, which happens most often during periods, but it can also happen at other times.

The symptoms of endometriosis vary. Some people experience mild symptoms, but others can have moderate to severe symptoms. The severity of the pain does not indicate the degree or stage of the condition. One can have a mild form of the disease yet experience agonizing pain. It is also possible to have a severe form and have very little discomfort.

The variable and broad symptoms of endometriosis mean that health care workers do not easily diagnose it, and many individuals suffering from it have limited awareness of the condition. This can cause a lengthy delay between onset of symptoms and diagnosis (1).

In the UK, the average interval between symptom onset and definitive diagnosis is 8 years (2). One-third of patients consulted their GP six or more times before receiving a diagnosis (3).

In some cases, endometriosis can be asymptomatic. Symptoms may vary from woman to woman, ranging from mild or moderate to severe.

Pelvic pain is the most common symptom of endometriosis.

Dysmenorrhea associated with endometriosis is dull or crampy pelvic pain that typically begins 1–2 days before the period, persists throughout the period and can continue for several days afterwards. Pelvic pain is typically chronic and described as dull, throbbing, sharp and/or burning. Pelvic pain or pressure are also the most common symptoms associated with adnexal mass.

DOI: 10.1201/9781032684819-5

A related observation is that some women transition between these categories, progressing from episodic and localized pain to that which is chronic, complex and more difficult to treat. Also, women with this disease that is anatomically severe can have minimal symptoms and women with minimal evidence of endometriosis can have severe life affecting symptoms (4).

Furthermore, endometriosis is challenging to diagnose because of the symptomatic overlap between the condition and other causes of pelvic pain, such as irritable bowel syndrome or pelvic inflammatory disease (PID) (4,5).

Symptoms associated with endometriosis vary and include a combination of the following (4,5):

- Chronic pelvic pain or low back pain
- Heavy menstrual bleeding or intermenstrual bleed
- Pain during and/or after sexual intercourse
- Lower back pain that may occur at any time during menstrual cycle
- Chronic fatigue
- Depression and or anxiety (depression is not a direct symptom but may be a side effect of the long diagnosis)
- Abdominal bloating, diarrhoea, constipation and nausea, especially during menstrual period, difficult or painful defecation
- Cyclical rectal bleed
- Haematuria
- Haemoptysis
- Painful micturition
- Painful caesarean section scar

In addition to the previous list, endometriosis can cause infertility. Infertility occurs due to the effects of endometriosis in the ovaries or fallopian tubes.

There is little correlation between the extent of endometrial lesions and severity or duration of symptoms: some individuals with visibly large lesions have mild symptoms, and others with few lesions have severe symptoms.

The symptoms of endometriosis tend to be cyclical—in many cases, symptoms start immediately before menstruation and cease as bleeding ends, becoming more chronic with ongoing unmanaged disease (4).

Teenagers who suffer with painful periods, experience fainting or collapse when having a period, or who miss school because of their period problems should be considered as possibly suffering from the condition.

Keeping a diary of these cyclical symptoms, including dysmenorrhoea; dysuria; and pain, straining or obstructed defecation, is a useful tool that can help with both diagnosis and assessment of treatment outcomes and is recommended by NICE as a measure to aid health care discussions (6).

Symptoms often improve after menopause, but in some cases, painful symptoms can persist. Chronic pain may be due to pain centres in the brain becoming hyper-responsive over time (central sensitization), which can occur at any point throughout the life-course of endometriosis, including treated, insufficiently treated and untreated endometriosis, and may persist even when endometriosis lesions are no longer visible.

Symptoms associated with different types of endometrioses:

- Women with peritoneal or deep-infiltrating endometriosis often present with dyspareunia. Deep-infiltrating endometriosis lesions can occur on the uterosacral and cardinal ligaments, pouch of Douglas, posterior vaginal fornix and anterior rectal wall (7)
- Introital or superficial dyspareunia can result from lesions of the cervix (8), hymen (9) and perineum (10)
- Women with bladder endometriosis typically present with nonspecific urinary symptoms of frequency, urgency and pain at micturition (11). Bladder symptoms get worse with menses. Ureteral endometriosis can be asymptomatic or can be associated with colicky flank pain or gross haematuria
- Women with endometriosis in the ureters can be asymptomatic or get colicky flank pain or gross haematuria
- Women with bowel endometriosis can suffer with diarrhoea, bowel cramps/pain, constipation, dyschezia and bowel cramping (12). Rectal bleeding may occur but is rare
- Women with deep-infiltrating endometriosis of the posterior cul-de-sac and rectovaginal septum typically present with dyspareunia and painful defecation (13)
- Women with thoracic endometriosis can present with chest pain, pneumothorax or haemothorax, haemoptysis or neck pain (14)
- Women with endometriosis of the abdominal wall typically present with a painful abdominal wall, and the pain can be cyclical with menstruation or continuous (15)

This means a patient with severe endometriosis can have mild symptoms and a patient with mild endometriosis can have severe symptoms.

Similar to other chronic pain conditions, women with endometriosis often report fatigue and depression.

Infertility is significantly more common in patients with endometriosis, with a doubling of risk compared with women without endometriosis (16). Endometriosis is found in 30–50% of women who present for assisted reproductive treatment (17).

The World Health Organization (WHO) recognizes the importance of endometriosis and its impact on people's sexual and reproductive health, quality of life and overall wellbeing (18).

WHO is partnering with multiple stakeholders, including academic institutions, non-state actors and other organizations that are actively involved in research, to identify effective models of endometriosis diagnosis, prevention, treatment and care (18). WHO recognizes the importance of advocating for increased awareness, policies and services for endometriosis and collaborates with civil society and endometriosis patient support groups in this regard. WHO is also collaborating with relevant stakeholders to facilitate and support the collection and analysis of country- and region-specific endometriosis prevalence data for decision-making.

ENDOMETRIOSIS-ASSOCIATED OR HIGH-RISK COMORBIDITIES

Endometriosis is a multisystem condition, perhaps because of common pathogenesis or as a consequence of the chronic endogenous response to the presence of endometriotic lesions. Although pelvic pain is the most common symptom of possible endometriosis, women with endometriosis also have a high risk of co-occurring or evolving multisite pain.

Irritable bowel syndrome is a common co-occurring diagnosis that reinforces the importance of awareness on endometriosis among gastroenterologists (19). These conditions may share a common cause; they may arise together owing to shared environmental or genetic factors, and/or the occurrence of comorbid pain conditions could be due to changes in pain perception after repeated sensitization.

Beyond access to an appropriate, skilled physician, the wide range of symptoms associated with endometriosis—many of which are stigmatized or normalized—reduces the likelihood of referral and increases time to referral to appropriate specialists.

Patients with endometriosis have a higher risk of presentation with fibromyalgia, rheumatoid arthritis, psoriatic arthritis and osteoarthritis (20).

Patients have a higher risk of migraine (21).

Nearly 50% of patients with bladder pain syndrome or interstitial cystitis have endometriosis (22).

Women with endometriosis have a greater risk of presenting with uterine fibroids and adenomyosis (23,24). They are also at greater risk of a subsequent diagnosis of malignancies, autoimmune diseases, early natural menopause and cerebrovascular and cardiovascular conditions.

Increased risk of ovarian cancer among women with endometriosis has been confirmed recently as well. A meta-analysis (25) found a nearly twofold greater relative risk of ovarian cancer among patients with endometriosis.

It is well-recognized that coexisting gynaecological conditions such as adenomyosis and uterine fibroids, as well as associations with endometrial cancer, can be influenced by diagnostic biases and failure to distinguish between diagnoses in women undergoing hysterectomy and those in women with an intact uterus. When attempting to infer a causal relation between endometriosis and other conditions, applying rigorous prospective temporality (rather than cross-sectional co-occurrence) is particularly important for valid subsequent risk associations. These studies need large study populations with well-documented data.

DIFFERENTIAL DIAGNOSIS

Endometriosis is challenging to diagnose because of overlap of symptoms between this condition and other causes of pelvic pain.

Non-Gynaecological Causes

- Irritable bowel syndrome (IBS)
- Appendicitis
- Renal colic, urinary tract infection (UTI)
- Constipation
- Diverticulitis
- Bowel obstruction
- Strangulated hernia
- Post-herpetic neuralgia

Gynaecological and Obstetrical Causes

- Pelvic inflammatory disease (PID)
- Ovarian cyst
- Rupture of corpus luteum cyst
- Ovulation
- Fibroid degeneration

- Pelvic cancer
- Adhesions due to previous surgery
- Miscarriage

SEVERITY OF SYMPTOMS RELATED TO ENDOMETRIOSIS CLASSIFICATION SYSTEMS

Several classification, staging and reporting systems have been developed; 22 systems were published between 1973 and 2021 (26). The three most commonly used systems are the revised American Society for Reproductive Medicine (rASRM) classification (stages I–IV; where stage I is equivalent to "minimal" disease and stage IV to "severe" disease), the ENZIAN (and newer #ENZIAN) classification, and the Endometriosis Fertility Index (EFI) (see Chapter 2).

> It is important to note that the presentation of symptoms does not necessarily correspond to the severity of the condition or progression of the condition.

Many validation studies and reports on the implementation of the different systems have been published. Unfortunately, no international agreement exists on how to describe endometriosis or how to classify it. As most systems show no, or very little, correlation with patients' symptoms and outcomes, this is further evidence of our lack of understanding of the physiology underlying the symptoms associated with endometriosis.

The bias in diagnosis itself may be influenced by variations in clinical symptoms among different populations not adequately captured or appreciated by standard clinical definitions or may represent implicit bias in health care, leading to an alternate interpretation of the same symptoms affecting the likelihood of diagnosis.

> The rASRM system (scored at surgery on the basis of the extent of visualized superficial peritoneal lesions, endometriomas and adhesions) has been shown to have poor correlation with pain, fertility outcomes and prognosis; and the ENZIAN system (which additionally includes deep endometriosis) has been shown to have poor correlation with symptoms and infertility.

Moreover, studies from African and Asian countries are considerably under-represented compared with European and North American countries.

MECHANISMS OF ENDOMETRIOSIS-ASSOCIATED PAIN

There are several theories on the causes of pain, which is the most common and debilitating symptom:

- The development of a new blood supply and associated nerves (neuroangiogenesis) is considered key to the establishment of endometriotic lesions and the activation of peripheral pain pathways
- Sensory C, sensory Ad, cholinergic and adrenergic nerve fibres have all been detected in lesions
- Oestrogens can promote crosstalk between immune cells and nerves within lesions, increasing expression of nociceptive ion channels such as the transient receptor potential cation channel subfamily V member 1 (27)
- Factors that promote inflammation and nerve growth, such as nerve growth factor, tumour necrosis factor α and interleukin 1-β, are increased in the peritoneal fluid of women with endometriosis and may exacerbate a neuroinflammatory cascade
- Consistent with other conditions associated with chronic pain, endometriosis is associated with unique, and sometimes disease-specific, alterations in the peripheral and central nervous systems, including changes in the volume of regions of the brain and in brain biochemistry (28)
- Increased risk of central sensitization may partially explain why approximately 30% of patients with endometriosis will develop chronic pelvic pain that is unresponsive to conventional treatments, including surgery (29)
- Among endometriosis patients with central sensitization, the removal of the endometriotic lesions is unlikely to result in adequate pain remediation owing to continued activation of the central nervous system (30)

Thus, endometriosis-associated pain does not neatly fall into one of the three main categories of chronic pain (that is, nociceptive, neuropathic or nociplastic) (31,32). For example, some patients have primarily nociceptive or neuropathic pain, others have primarily nociplastic pain, and the rest have a mixed phenotype with variable contributions of nociceptive, neuropathic and nociplastic pain.

RED FLAG SIGNS

The diagnosis of endometriosis should be considered in women (including girls aged 17 and under) presenting with one (or more) of the these symptoms or signs: chronic pelvic pain with or without cyclic flares, dysmenorrhea (affecting daily activities and quality of life), deep dyspareunia, cyclical gastrointestinal symptoms (particularly dyschezia), cyclical urinary symptoms (particularly haematuria or dysuria) or infertility in association with one (or more) of the preceding symptoms or signs. With any of the following symptoms or signs, urgent admission or assessment is needed:

- Shoulder tip pain (pain under the shoulder blade)
- Pneumothorax
- Cyclical cough/Haemoptysis/Chest pain
- Cyclical scar swelling/Pain
- Extreme fatigue

NICE GUIDELINES FOR ENDOMETRIOSIS: DIAGNOSIS AND MANAGEMENT (6)

Guidance from NICE suggests to suspect endometriosis in women, including young women aged 17 and under, presenting with one or more of the following symptoms and signs:

- Chronic pelvic pain
- Period-related pain (dysmenorrhoea) affecting daily activities and quality of life
- Deep pain during or after sexual intercourse
- Period-related or cyclical gastrointestinal symptoms, in particular painful bowel movements
- Period-related or cyclical urinary symptoms, in particular blood in the urine or pain passing urine
- Infertility in association with one or more of the previous symptoms

KEY POINT SUMMARY

- Endometriosis is a chronic disease associated with life-impacting pain during periods, sexual intercourse, bowel movements and/or urination; chronic pelvic pain; abdominal bloating; nausea; fatigue; and sometimes depression, anxiety and infertility.

- Clinical presentation is variable with some women experiencing several severe symptoms and others having no symptoms at all.
- Consider endometriosis when women of reproductive age present with abdominal-pelvic pain associated with menstruation, urination, defecation and sexual intercourse and/or infertility.

REFERENCES

1. Agarwal SK, Chapron C, Giudice LC, et al. Clinical diagnosis of endometriosis: A call to action. *Am J Obstet Gynecol* 2019;4:354–64.
2. All Party Parliamentary Group on Endometriosis, Endometriosis UK. *Endometriosis in the UK: Time for change.* London: Endometriosis UK, 2020. www.endometriosis-uk.org/sites/default/files/files/Endometriosis%20 APPG%20Report%20Oct%202020.pdf (accessed 25 Aug 2023).
3. Pugsley Z, Ballard K. Management of endometriosis in general practice: The pathway to diagnosis. *Br J Gen Pract* 2007;57(539):470–6.
4. Saunders P, Horne A. Endometriosis: Etiology, pathobiology, and therapeutic prospects. *Cell* 2021;184(11):2807–24.
5. Foti P, Farina R, Palmucci S, et al. Endometriosis: Clinical features, MR imaging findings and pathologic correlation. *Insights Imaging* 2018; 9(2):149–72.
6. NICE. *Endometriosis: Diagnosis and management.* NICE Guideline 73. NICE, 2017. www.nice.org.uk/ng73 (accessed 25 Aug 2023).
7. Vercellini P, Fedele L, Aimi G, et al. Association between endometriosis stage, lesion type, patient characteristics and severity of pelvic pain symptoms: A multivariate analysis of over 1000 patients. *Hum Reprod* 2007;22:266.
8. Wang S, Li XC, Lang JH. Cervical endometriosis: Clinical character and management experience in a 27-year span. *Am J Obstet Gynecol* 2011;205:452.e 1.
9. Canlorbe G, Laas E, Cortez A, et al. Spontaneous hymeneal endometriosis: 1 rare cause of dyspareunia. *BMJ Case Rep* 2014;2014.
10. Nasu K, Okamoto M, Nishida M, et al. Endometriosis of the perinuem. *J Obstet Gynecol Res* 2013;39:1095.
11. Berlanda N, Vercellini P, Carmignani L, et al. Ureteral and vesical endometriosis. Two different clinical entities sharing the same pathogenesis. *Obstet Gynecol Surv* 2009;64:830.
12. Ballard K, Lane H, Hudelist G, et al. Can specific pain symptoms help in the diagnosis of endometriosis? A cohort study of women with chronic pelvic pain. *Fertil Steril* 2010;94:20.
13. Porpora MG, Koninckx PR, Piazze J, et al. Correlation between endometriosis and pelvic pain. *J Am Assoc Gynecol Laparosc* 1999;6:429.
14. Rousset P, Gregory J, Rousset-Jablonski C, et al. MR diagnosis of diaphragmatic endometriosis. *Eur Radiol* 2016;26:3968.
15. Horton JD, Dezee KJ, Ahnfeldt EP, et al. Abdominal wall endometriosis: A surgeon's perspective and review of 445 cases. *Am J Surg* 2008; 196:207.
16. Prescott J, Farland LV, Tobias DK, et al. A prospective cohort study of endometriosis and subsequent risk of infertility. *Hum Reprod* 2016;31:1475–82. doi:10.1093/humrep/dew085

17. Eskenazi B, Warner ML. Epidemiology of endometriosis epidemiology of endometriosis. *Obstet Gynecol Clin North Am* 1997;24:235–58. doi:10. 1016/S0889-8545(05)70302-8 pmid:9163765
18. World Health Organization (WHO). *International classification of diseases, 11th revision (ICD-11)*. Geneva: WHO, 2018.
19. DiVasta AD, Zimmerman LA, Vitonis AF, et al. Overlap between irritable bowel syndrome diagnosis and endometriosis in adolescents. *Clin Gastroenterol Hepatol* 2021;19:528–37.
20. Larrosa Pardo F, Bondesson E, Schelin MEC. A diagnosis of rheumatoid arthritis, endometriosis or IBD is associated with later onset of fibromyalgia and chronic widespread pain. *Eur J Pain* 2019;23:1563–73.
21. Jenabi E, Khazaei S. Endometriosis and migraine headache risk: A meta-analysis. *Women Health* 2020;60:939–45.
22. Rodríguez MA, Afari N, Buchwald DS. National Institute of Diabetes and Digestive and Kidney Diseases Working Group on Urological Chronic Pelvic Pain. Evidence for overlap between urological and nonurological unexplained clinical conditions. *J Urol* 2009;182:2123–31.
23. Gallagher CS, Mäkinen N, Harris HR, et al. Genome-wide association and epidemiological analyses reveal common genetic origins between uterine leiomyomata and endometriosis. *Nat Commun* 2019;10:4857.
24. Upson K, Missmer SA. Epidemiology of Adenomyosis. *Semin Reprod Med* 2020;38:89–107.
25. Kvaskoff M, Mahamat-Saleh Y, Farland LV, et al. Endometriosis and cancer: A systematic review and meta-analysis. *Hum Reprod Update* 2021;27:393–420.
26. Vermeulen N, Abrao MS, Einarsson JI, et al. International working group of AAGL, ESGE, ESHRE and WES. Endometriosis classification, staging and reporting systems: A review on the road to a universally accepted endometriosis classification. *Hum Reprod Open* 2021;2021:hoab025. doi:10.1093/hropen/hoab025 pmid:34693032
27. Greaves E, Temp J, Esnal-Zufiurre A, et al. Estradiol is a critical mediator of macrophage-nerve cross talk in peritoneal endometriosis. *Am J Pathol* 2015;185:2286–97. doi:10.1016/j.ajpath.2015.04.012 pmid:26073038
28. As-Sanie S, Harris RE, Napadow V, et al. Changes in regional gray matter volume in women with chronic pelvic pain: A voxel-based morphometry study. *Pain* 2012;153:1006–14. doi:10.1016/j.pain.2012.01.032 pmid: 22387096
29. Coccia ME, Rizzello F, Palagiano A, et al. Long-term follow-up after laparoscopic treatment for endometriosis: Multivariate analysis of predictive factors for recurrence of endometriotic lesions and pain. *Eur J Obstet Gynecol Reprod Biol* 2011;157:78–83. doi:10.1016/j.ejogrb.2011.02.008 pmid:21481523
30. Stratton P, Khachikyan I, Sinaii N, et al. Association of chronic pelvic pain and endometriosis with signs of sensitization and myofascial pain. *Obstet Gynecol* 2015;125:719–28. doi:10.1097/AOG.0000000000000663 pmid:25730237
31. Cohen SP, Vase L, Hooten WM. Chronic pain: An update on burden, best practices, and new advances. *Lancet* 2021;397:2082–97. doi:10.1016/ S0140-6736(21)00393-7 pmid:34062143
32. Lamvu G, Carrillo J, Ouyang C, et al. Chronic pelvic pain in women: A review. *JAMA* 2021;325:2381–91. doi:10.1001/jama.2021.2631 pmid:34128995 [CrossRef] [PubMed] [Google Scholar]

FURTHER READING

All Party Parliamentary Group on Endometriosis, Endometriosis UK. *Endometriosis in the UK: Time for change*. London: Endometriosis UK, 2020. www.endometriosis-uk.org/sites/default/files/files/Endometriosis%20APPG%20Report%20Oct%202020.pdf (accessed 20 Aug 2023).

pcwhf.co.uk/wp-content/uploads/2022/05/HLHH_Spring21_toptipsendo.pdf (accessed 25 Aug 2023).

Primary Care Women's Health Forum. *10 top tips for endometriosis management in primary care*. Arlesey: PCWHF, 2021. Available at: pcwhf.co.uk/resources/10-top-tips-for-endometriosis-management-in-primary-care/

CHAPTER 6

Investigations

....

The variable and broad symptoms of endometriosis mean that health care workers do not easily diagnose it, and many individuals suffering from it have limited awareness of the condition. This can cause a lengthy delay between onset of symptoms and diagnosis (1).

A careful history of menstrual symptoms and chronic pelvic pain provides the basis for suspecting endometriosis. Although several screening tools and tests have been proposed and tested, none are currently validated to accurately identify or predict individuals or populations that are most likely to have the disease.

PELVIC EXAMINATION

Although clinical examination may be normal in women with minimal–mild endometriosis, abnormal findings, such as a retroverted uterus (RV) with reduced mobility, painful rectovaginal or uterosacral nodules or the presence of adnexal masses, are not rare in advanced endometriosis. Umbilical, abdominal or episiotomy scar nodules may easily be detected, particularly at the time of menses. Pelvic floor spasm might also be present. While physical examination findings are helpful, the examination can also be normal.

Clinicians must offer an abdominal and pelvic examination to women with suspected endometriosis as per NICE Guidelines (2). The Primary Care Women's Health Forum (PCWHF) also recommends considering sexual health screening, when appropriate, for women with suspected endometriosis (3).

DOI: 10.1201/9781032684819-6

NICE stresses that a normal examination does not exclude the possibility of endometriosis (4). A pelvic examination should only be offered when appropriate (4), and it is most useful when there is a need to exclude alternative diagnosis as such pelvic inflammatory disease.

BLOOD TESTS

There are no abnormal laboratory blood tests for diagnosing endometriosis. While several urinary and endometrial biomarkers have been studied for the non-invasive diagnosis of disease, none are clinically useful (5,6).

Serum CA125

Serum cancer antigen CA125 can be elevated in women with endometriosis (i.e., greater than 35 units/mL), but the role of serum CA125 in primary diagnosis of endometriosis is undefined. Serum CA125 should not be routinely ordered in women with suspected endometriosis because other diseases notably ovarian cancer also elevate CA125 (7,8).

Although it is an active area of research, there are no biomarkers with adequate specificity or sensitivity to identify endometriosis (9,10) (including CA125), according to NICE (4) and the European Society of Human Reproduction and Embryology (ESHRE) (11).

Other Blood Tests

If patient is admitted with pelvic pain, one must do baseline blood tests (i.e., full blood count, urea and electrolytes and C-reactive protein): White cells may be raised in appendicitis or pelvis inflammatory disease. Other differential diagnoses of acute pain are ectopic pregnancy, torsion of an ovarian cyst, primary dysmenorrhoea and irritable bowel syndrome (IBS).

Urine Pregnancy Test or beta-hCG

Perform this test on all women of reproductive age to rule out pregnancy.

ULTRASOUND SCANS

Ultrasonography and magnetic resonance imaging (ideally two dimensional, T2-weighted sequences without fat suppression) can be used to diagnose endometriosis preoperatively, but the absence of findings on imaging does not exclude endometriosis, particularly superficial perito-neal disease (13).

Transvaginal Ultrasound Scan (TVUS)

Transvaginal ultrasound (TVU) is evolving as an essential tool in the workup for women with pelvic pain and suspected endometriosis. Several studies have demonstrated the accuracy and reliability of TVU for the diagnosis of pelvic deep-infiltrating endometriosis and pouch of Douglas obliteration. Assessment of the anterior pelvic compartment for urinary DIE and uterovesical adhesions should also be considered in the transvaginal ultrasound examination for women with pelvic pain sus-pected endometriosis. In addition, the use of ultrasound markers such as ovarian endometriomas and ovarian immobility may also aid in the assessment for disease severity.

NICE recommends transvaginal ultrasound scanning as a first line for the investigation of endometriosis. The ability to map disease location and extent preoperatively allows for appropriate triaging, surgical plan-ning, patient counselling, and, in turn, improved care for women with severe endometriosis.

It is important to detail the symptoms, specifying the likely diagno-sis of endometriosis when referring for a scan. This will prompt sonog-raphers to look more specifically for endometriotic deposits. This is important to investigate suspected endometriosis even if pelvic and/or abdominal examination is normal and to identify endometriomas and deep endometriosis involving bladder, ureter or bowel. If deep-infiltrating endometriosis is found on ultrasound, the scan should be extended to include an assessment of the kidneys to rule out hydronephrosis.

Transvaginal ultrasound scan is often normal in those who are sub-sequently diagnosed with superficial or deep endometriosis; however, it can reliably identify those with endometriomas and exclude differentials such as non-endometriotic cysts and adenomyosis.

Transvaginal ultrasound has the ability to dynamically assess mobility and site-specific tenderness, known as "soft markers," for endometriosis, suggestive of superficial disease and pelvic adhesions. The loss of the sliding sign on transvaginal ultrasound assessment indicates obliteration of the pouch of Douglas (14), which is an essential piece of information to obtain for surgical planning.

Nodules of endometriosis tend to appear sonographically as solid, hypoechoic, irregular masses. They may contain echogenic foci or small cystic spaces and often show little or no blood flow on colour Doppler.

Advanced TVUS

Advanced TVUS specialists might assess for subtle features of endometriosis such as loss of mobility of the ovaries and within the pouch of Douglas (7); site-specific tenderness and nodularity (a sensitivity of 79% and specificity of 94%) have been reported with experienced sonographers (12).

Sensitivity of 3D ultrasound for deep endometriosis is 87% (13,15).

However, access to specialist ultrasonography is limited in most settings. When TVUS is declined, inappropriate or unavailable, offer transabdominal ultrasound (although sensitivity and specificity is lower) (4).

Transabdominal Ultrasound Scan

Transabdominal scanning is of a very limited use in the assessment of endometriosis beyond the detection of ovarian endometrioma. However, a good quality transabdominal scan can reveal deep endometriosis affective bladder and bowel with similar sensitivity to MRI.

If transvaginal scan is not appropriate or refused by patient, a transabdominal ultrasound scan of the pelvis is an alternative option (3). A transabdominal scan has a lower diagnostic sensitivity (4).

Although a normal ultrasound scan indicates the absence of endometriomas, it does not exclude the possibility of endometriosis in general (2), as endometriotic deposits are hard to detect using this method.

Contrast-Enhanced Ultrasound Scan (CEUS)

Endometriotic implants present a variable contrast enhancement and can appear as lesions with homogeneous or heterogeneous enhancement with a non-enhanced centre, depending on the associated fibrotic component. It is important to remember that ultrasound contrast agent (sulphur hexafluorid microbubbles, Sonovue) is purely intravascular (unlike iodine or gadolinium-based contrast, which has an interstitial phase), so an enhancing lesion in the CEUS reflects a vascularized lesion (16). Thus, the fibrotic areas will not present contrast enhancement.

The use of contrast-enhanced ultrasound in deep pelvic endometriosis can be useful to assess the preservation of the layered structure of the intestinal wall (differentiating it from intestinal neoplasia), to define the extension and morphology of the implant and to assess an extrinsic origin in cases of ureteric involvement (differentiating it from urothelial neoplasia). In cases of deep endometriosis compressing the ureter or causing hydronephrosis, CEUS can also be helpful to assess if an enhancing lesion in the ureter has an intraluminal (as seen in urothelial neoplasms) or an extraluminal origin (as seen in endometriotic implants) (16).

MRI

A typical pelvic MRI lasts 30 to 60 minutes. The initial results from an MRI scan may come within a few days, but your comprehensive results can take up to a week or more. The magnetic field generated by the MRI temporarily aligns the water molecules in the body. Radio waves take these aligned particles and produce faint signals, which the machine then records as images. The magnets used in an MRI can cause problems with pacemakers so make sure before referring the patient. If the patient is claustrophobic, she may feel uncomfortable while in the MRI machine. It may be a good idea to prescribe a low-dose anxiolytic.

Ovarian and deep endometriosis may be visible on magnetic resonance imaging (MRI), but a normal MRI does not exclude endometriosis (13):

- Do not use pelvic MRI as the primary investigation to diagnose endometriosis in women with signs or symptoms suggestive of endometriosis (2)
- Consider pelvic MRI to assess the extent of deep endometriosis involving bowel, bladder or ureter (2). Patient can be referred for cystoscopy if bladder involvement is suspected
- Ensure that pelvic MRI scans are interpreted by a health care professional with specialist expertise in gynaecological imaging

Limitations of MRI

Despite all the advantages of MRI over all other imaging modalities, it, nonetheless, has several limitations, including:

- Non-pigmented lesions will not be hyperintense on T1 and thus will be harder to detect
- Small foci may have variable signal intensity
  - May appear similar to normal endometrium: low T1, high T2
  - Hypointense on all sequences
  - Hyperintense on all sequences (17)
- Plaque-like implants are difficult to delineate (18)
- Adhesions cannot be directly identified, usually relying on the distortion of normal anatomy to imply their existence (18)

Saline Infusion SonoPODography (SISP)

Women with infertility are often investigated with saline infusion sono-hysterography and hysterosalpingo-contrast sonography. The high prevalence of endometriosis in this population also warrants an evaluation with transvaginal ultrasound for deep endometriosis. In most patients, the fluid infused to assess the cavity and tubal patency spilled through patent tubes and filled the pouch of Douglas (POD), yielding a "stand-off" view of posterior compartment structures, including uterosacral ligaments, rectovaginal septum and the pouch of Douglas.

This is a novel technique that may be able to diagnose superficial peritoneal endometriosis on ultrasonography although it needs to be validated (19).

LAPAROSCOPY WITH HISTOLOGICAL CONFIRMATION

In patients with suspected endometriosis in whom imaging has shown no obvious pelvic pathology or for whom empirical treatment has been unsuccessful, laparoscopy is recommended for diagnosis.

Laparoscopic visualization is the gold standard investigation, unless visible lesions are seen in the posterior vaginal fornix (4).

Diagnostic laparoscopy enables direct visualization of any endometriotic deposits; however, it is invasive, involves small risk of major complications (bowel perforation) and is not chosen or indicated in every case (20).

Consider Laparoscopy (2)

- To diagnose endometriosis in women with suspected endometriosis even if ultrasound scan (USS) is normal
- For women with suspected deep endometriosis involving bladder, ureter or bowel, consider pelvic USS or MRI before an operative laparoscopy
- It should be performed by a gynaecologist with specialist skills and training in endometriosis
- During a diagnostic laparoscopy, consider taking a biopsy of suspected lesion
- Negative histological result does not exclude endometriosis

Laparoscopy for endometriosis should always involve a comprehensive exploration of the abdominal and pelvic contents. However, it is an invasive diagnostic tool with potential morbidity. There is often a delay between symptoms and referral for laparoscopy, which could be due to lack of knowledge among health care professionals and inadequate use of diagnostic tools.

Histopathological confirmation is ideal; however, histologic definitions for endometriosis have remained stagnant for decades, with a lower-than-expected sensitivity (21), particularly among younger women with endometriosis. Superficial peritoneal endometriosis has been described as having a black (powder burn) or dark bluish appearance from the accumulation of blood pigments. However, lesions can appear as white opacifications, red flame-like lesions, or yellow-brown patches in earlier, active stages of disease.

Ovarian endometriomas, classically described as "chocolate cysts," contain old menstrual blood, necrotic fluid and other poorly defined components that give their contents a dark brown appearance. Adhesions are often found in association with endometriomas and consist of fibrous scar tissue resulting from chronic inflammation.

Almost 40% of laparoscopies done for pelvic pain do not identify any pathology (22). Clinicians should always consider other pelvic and non-pelvic visceral and somatic structures, as well as centrally mediated pain factors, that could be generating or contributing to the pain (22).

NICE and ESHRE guidance suggests that laparoscopy with histology is the gold standard for diagnosis (2,11); however, many researchers and clinicians believe that clinical and radiographical features (as described before) are sufficient for diagnosis, particularly for ovarian and deep subtypes.

Similarly, some guidelines (including those from ESHRE) suggest that laparoscopy may not be indicated for patients with symptoms controlled by medical treatment if the patient agrees with a working diagnosis of endometriosis.

If a full systematic laparoscopy is performed and is normal, woman can be reassured that she does not have endometriosis.

RED FLAG SIGNS

The diagnosis of endometriosis should be considered in women (including girls aged 17 and under) presenting with one (or more) of the following symptoms or signs:

- Chronic pelvic pain with or without cyclic flares
- Dysmenorrhea (affecting daily activities and quality of life)
- Deep dyspareunia
- Cyclical gastrointestinal symptoms (particularly dyschezia)
- Cyclical urinary symptoms (particularly haematuria or dysuria)

- Infertility in association with one (or more) of the preceding symptoms or signs (23)
- Shoulder tip pain (pain under the shoulder blade)
- Catamenial pneumothorax, cyclical cough/haemoptysis/chest pain
- Cyclical scar swelling/pain can indicate endometriosis at extra-abdominal sites (24)
- Fatigue (commonly reported by women with endometriosis)

An abdominal-pelvic examination may help to identify ovarian and deep disease (25).

If the patient is admitted with pelvic pain, one must do:

- Baseline blood tests (FBC, U&Es, CRP): White cells may be raised in appendicitis or pelvis inflammatory disease
- Urine pregnancy test or beta-hCG on all women of reproductive age to rule out pregnancy

"Working Diagnosis" of Probable Endometriosis

In women with a high suspicion of endometriosis, in whom imaging has not shown obvious pelvic pathology and a laparoscopy has not been done or is awaited, giving a "working diagnosis" of probable endometriosis and instigating early medical treatment without waiting for a more definitive diagnosis can be helpful (1,26). This is an emerging concept for which some people use the terms "working" and "clinical" diagnosis interchangeably.

KEY POINT SUMMARY

- Clinical diagnosis is difficult, partly because the symptoms are often non-specific and may be attributed to other conditions, for example, irritable bowel syndrome, or misdiagnosed as functional or psychosomatic (27,28).
- Clinicians must offer an abdominal and pelvic examination including per speculum examination to women with suspected endometriosis. Consider sexual health screening as recommended by Primary Care Women's Health Forum (PCWHF).
- No need to do routine CA125. A raised serum CA125 (35 IU/mL or more) may be consistent with having endometriosis. However, endometriosis may be present despite a normal CA125 (less than 35 IU/mL).
- Diagnose endometriosis in women with suspected endometriosis even if USS is normal.

- If a transvaginal scan is not appropriate, consider a transabdominal scan of the pelvis.
- For women with suspected deep endometriosis involving bladder, ureter or bowel, consider pelvic USS or MRI before an operative laparoscopy.
- Operative laparoscopy should be performed by a gynaecologist with specialist skills and training in endometriosis.
- During a diagnostic laparoscopy, consider taking a biopsy of suspected lesion.

REFERENCES

1. Agarwal SK, Chapron C, Giudice LC, et al. Clinical diagnosis of endometriosis: A call to action. *Am J Obstet Gynecol* 2019;4:354–64.
2. NICE. *Endometriosis: When should I suspect endometriosis?* NICE Clinical Knowledge Summary. cks.nice.org.uk/topics/endometriosis/diagnosis/when-to-suspect-endometriosis (accessed 12 Aug 2023).
3. Primary Care Women's Health Forum. *10 top tips for endometriosis management in primary care.* Arlesey: PCWHF, 2021. pcwhf.co.uk/wp-content/uploads/2022/05/HLHH_Spring21_toptipsendo.pdf (accessed 12 Aug 2023).
4. NICE. *Endometriosis: Diagnosis and management.* NICE Guideline 73. NICE, 2017. www.nice.org.uk/ng73 (accessed 18 Feb 2023).
5. Liu E, Nisenblat V, Farquhar C, et al. Urinary biomarkers for the non-invasive diagnosis of endometriosis. *Cochrane Database Syst Rev* 2015:CD012019.
6. Gupta D, Hull ML, Fraser I, et al. Endometrial biomarkers for the non-invasive diagnosis of endometriosis. *Cochrane Database Syst Rev* 2016;4:CD012165.
7. Cheng YM, Wang ST, Chou CY. Serum CA-125 in preoperative patients at high risk for endometriosis. *Obstet Gynecol* 2002;99:375.
8. Mol BW, Bayram N, Lijmer JG, et al. The performance of CA125 measurement in the detection of endometriosis: A meta-analysis. *Fertil Steril* 1998;70:1101.
9. Nisenblat V, Bossuyt PMM, Shaikh R, et al. Blood biomarkers for the non-invasive diagnosis of endometriosis. *Cochrane Database Syst Rev* 2016;5:CD012179. doi:10.1002/14651858.CD012179 pmid:27132058 [CrossRef] [PubMed] [Google Scholar]
10. Tian Z, Chang XH, Zhao Y, et al. Current biomarkers for the detection of endometriosis. *Chin Med J (Engl)* 2020;133:2346–52. doi:10.1097/CM9.0000000000001063 pmid:32858595 [CrossRef] [PubMed] [Google Scholar]
11. Becker CM, Bokor A, Heikinheimo O. ESHRE guideline: Endometriosis. *Hum Reprod Open* 2022;2022:hoac009. [CrossRef] [PubMed] [Google Scholar]
12. Guerriero S, Condous G, van den Bosch T, et al. Systematic approach to sonographic evaluation of the pelvis in women with suspected endometriosis, including terms, definitions, and measurements: A consensus opinion from the International Deep Endometriosis Analysis (IDEA) group. *Ultrasound Obstet Gynecol* 2016;48:318–32.

13. Nisenblat V, Bossuyt PMM, Farquhar C, et al. Imaging modalities for the non-invasive diagnosis of endometriosis. *Cochrane Database Syst Rev* 2016;2:CD009591. doi:10.1002/14651858.CD009591.pub2 pmid: 26919512 [CrossRef] [PubMed] [Google Scholar]

14. Reid S, Condous G. Transvaginal sonographic sliding sign: Accurate prediction of pouch of Douglas obliteration. *Ultrasound Obstet Gynecol* 2013;41(6):605. doi:10.1002/uog.12469-Pubmed

15. Guerriero S, Saba L, Ajossa S, et al. Three-dimensional ultrasonography in the diagnosis of deep endometriosis. *Hum Reprod* 2014;29:1189–98. doi:10.1093/humrep/deu054 pmid:24664128 [CrossRef] [PubMed] [Google Scholar]

16. Salvador J, Lorente E, Ripollés T, et al. Infiltrating endometriosis: Diagnostic keys in abdominal ultrasonography. *Radiología* 2020;62(6). doi:10.1016/j. rx.2020.09.007

17. Woodward PJ, Sohaey R, Mezzetti TP. Endometriosis: Radiologic-pathologic correlation. *Radiographics* 2001;21(1):193–216. Radiographics (full text)—Pubmed citation

18. Zawin M, Mccarthy S, Scoutt L, et al. Endometriosis: Appearance and detection at MR imaging. *Radiology* 1989;171(3):693–6. Radiology (abstract)—Pubmed citation

19. Leonardi M, Espada M, Lu C, et al. A novel ultrasound technique called saline infusion SonoPODography to visualize and understand the pouch of Douglas and posterior compartment contents: A feasibility study. *J Ultrasound Med* 2019;38:3301–9. doi:10.1002/jum.15022 pmid:31090229 [CrossRef] [PubMed] [Google Scholar]

20. Royal College of Obstetricians & Gynaecologists. *Diagnostic laparoscopy consent advice no. 2*. London: RCOG, 2017. www.rcog.org.uk/media/c5ycf 03i/diagnostic-laparoscopy-consent-advice-2.pdf (accessed 18 Feb 2023).

21. Taylor HS, Adamson GD, Diamond MP, et al. An evidence-based approach to assessing surgical versus clinical diagnosis of symptomatic endometriosis. *Int J Gynaecol Obstet* 2018;142:131–42. doi:10.1002/ijgo.12521 pmid:29729099

22. Lamvu G, Carrillo J, Ouyang C, et al. Chronic pelvic pain in women: A review. *JAMA* 2021;325:2381–91. doi:10.1001/jama.2021.2631 pmid: 34128995 [CrossRef] [PubMed] [Google Scholar]

23. Kuznetsov L, Dworzynski K, Davies M, et al. Diagnosis and management of endometriosis: Summary of NICE guidance. *BMJ* 2017;358:j3935. doi:10.1136/bmj.j3935 pmid:28877898 [FREE Full Text] [Google Scholar]

24. Levine D, Brown DL, Andreotti RF, et al. Management of asymptomatic ovarian and other adnexal cysts imaged at US: Society of Radiologists in Ultrasound consensus conference statement. *Radiology* 2010;256:943–54. doi:10.1148/radiol.10100213 pmid:20505067 [CrossRef] [PubMed] [Google Scholar]

25. Bazot M, Lafont C, Rouzier R, et al. Diagnostic accuracy of physical examination, transvaginal sonography, rectal endoscopic sonography, and magnetic resonance imaging to diagnose deep infiltrating endometriosis. *Fertil Steril* 2009;92:1825–33. doi:10.1016/j.fertnstert.2008.09.005 pmid:19019357 [CrossRef] [PubMed] [Google Scholar]

26. Jones R, Barraclough K, Dowrick C. When no diagnostic label is applied. *BMJ* 2010;340:c2683. doi:10.1136/bmj.c2683 pmid:20501578 [FREE Full Text] [Google Scholar]

27. Staal AHJ, van der Zanden M, Nap AW. Diagnostic delay of endometriosis in the Netherlands. *Gynecol Obstet Invest* 2016;81:321–4. doi:10.1159/000441911 pmid:26742108

28. Ballard KD, Seaman HE, de Vries CS, et al. Can symptomatology help in the diagnosis of endometriosis? Findings from a national case-control study—Part 1. *BJOG* 2008;115:1382–91. doi:10.1111/j.1471-0528.2008.01878.x pmid:18715240 [CrossRef] [PubMed] [Web of Science] [Google Scholar]

FURTHER READING

All Party Parliamentary Group on Endometriosis, Endometriosis UK. *Endometriosis in the UK: Time for change.* London: Endometriosis UK, 2020. www.endometriosis-uk.org/sites/default/files/files/Endometriosis%20APPG%20Report%20Oct%202020.pdf (accessed 18 Aug 2023).

Radiopedia.org/articles/endometriosis

RCOG. *The investigation and management of endometriosis.* Royal College of Obstetricians and Gynaecologists. 2006.

Royal College of Obstetricians and Gynaecologists. *Diagnostic laparoscopy consent advice no. 2.* London: RCOG, 2017. www.rcog.org.uk/media/c5ycf03i/diagnostic-laparoscopy-consent-advice-2.pdf (accessed 18 Aug 2023).

www.nice.org.uk/guidance/ng73

CHAPTER 7

Pharmacological Management

....

Drug treatment is used in women suffering with endometriosis in their reproductive years. The goal of pharmacological treatment is to reduce or eliminate pain, inhibit further development and regression of endometrial foci and restore fertility.

NICE recommends an initial 3-month trial of paracetamol or nonsteroidal anti-inflammatory drugs (NSAIDs) alone or with a combined oral contraceptive (COC) pill or continuous progestogen. This should be started in primary care if pain is suggestive of endometriosis (1,2). Initiation of pharmacological treatment of endometriosis can be done based on a clinical examination without the need to confirm the diagnosis by laparoscopy.

Pharmacotherapy may be part of the preparation for surgery as well as a complementary procedure in the postoperative period.

Women who do not want surgical treatment but who are experiencing mild-to-moderate symptoms, with no suggestion of an endometrioma, may be indicated for medical therapy (3). A review should be carried out after 3–6 months, or earlier if requested (3). Review appointments in primary care are opportunities to assess the outcomes of any treatment and consider further actions.

MEDICAL THERAPIES: NON-HORMONAL

Analgesia

Analgesics are the treatment option, particularly if hormonal treatments are not suitable or contraindicated or patient not keen to take it. They are used to reduce pain rather than to treat the condition itself. Simple

DOI: 10.1201/9781032684819-7

TABLE 7.1   Non-Hormonal Treatments

Treatment	Route	Side Effects	Comments
ANALGESICS OR NSAIDs	Oral	• Nausea, Indigestion • Loose stools • Headaches	Initial 3/12 trial period of paracetamol or NSAID alone or with COC or continuous progestogen
TRICYCLIC ANTIDEPRESSANTS (amitriptyline, nortriptyline)	Oral	• Weight gain • Constipation • Dizziness • Headaches Somnolence	
SSRI (for example, duloxetine) and ANTICONVULSANTS (for example, gabapentin and pregabalin)		• Dizziness • Blurred Vision • Constipation • Diarrhoea • Dry mouth • Difficulty sleeping	**www.nice.org.uk/ cg173**
PELVIC PHYSIO	See Chapter 8		**Women's health or pelvic health physiotherapy is not included in the NICE Guidelines for endometriosis**; however, it is included in the NICE Guidelines for chronic pelvic pain

analgesics such a paracetamol (4), co-codamol and codydramol can be used on PRN basis. It is important to discuss the side effects and benefits of analgesics taking in to account her preferences.

However, it is not a good idea to issue tramadol or morphine because of side effects and risk of addiction.

Nonsteroidal Anti-Inflammatory Drugs (NSAIDs)

Most women with suspected or known endometriosis use over-the-counter nonsteroidal anti-inflammatory drugs (NSAIDs). However, the available evidence to support their use is scarce. The data on the benefit of NSAIDs are limited to one small randomized control trial (RCT) (5).

They can be useful as "breakthrough medication" in the management of a pain flare.

But these are generally more effective if started prior to the menstruation and continuing throughout the period to gain maximum benefit. If prescribing an NSAID, make sure to exclude the contraindications and add PPI for gastric protection.

Nonsteroidal anti-inflammatory drugs inhibit the synthesis of prostaglandins, contribute to reducing the inflammatory process and resolve pain (6).

Neuromodulators

If the previous treatments are not effective and patient has complex pain with neuropathic symptoms, neuromodulators can be prescribed as per NICE Guidelines on Neuropathic Drugs CG 173 (1,6,7).

The most commonly used are analgesic tricyclic antidepressants (for example, amitriptyline, nortriptyline); selective serotonin uptake inhibitors (for example, duloxetine); and anticonvulsants (for example, gabapentin and pregabalin).

There is not strong evidence that these drugs manage endometriosis-associated pain (8).

These neuromodulators differ from conventional analgesics, such as NSAIDs, in that they primarily affect the central nervous system's modulation of pain rather than peripheral mediators of inflammation.

However, in a recent RCT for the management of chronic pelvic pain, gabapentin was not shown to be superior to placebo and was associated with dose-limiting side effects (8,9).

MEDICAL THERAPIES: HORMONAL

Hormone treatments for endometriosis include combined contraceptives, progestogens, gonadotrophin-releasing hormone (GnRH) agonists, GnRH antagonists and aromatase inhibitors (Table 7.2). Hormonal treatments for endometriosis focus on either lowering oestrogen or increasing progesterone to alter hormonal environments that promote endometriosis. The use of hormonal treatments, with the ambition of inducing amenorrhoea to reduce the negative effects of endometriosis, is a central aspect of endometriosis care (1,10,11).

Most of the currently used hormonal management is not suitable for persons suffering from endometriosis who wish to get pregnant, since they affect ovulation (1). The choice of treatment depends on effectiveness in the individual, adverse side effects, long-term safety, costs and availability.

TABLE 7.2 Hormonal Treatment

Treatment	Route	Side Effects	Comments
COMBINED CONTRACEPTIVE	• Oral (COC) • Patch • Vaginal ring	Nausea, headaches, breast tenderness, bloated feeling, breakthrough bleeding, increased risk of VTE	• Offer continuous COC if patient prefers amenorrhoea. • Continuous COC use may be superior to cyclical use for period pain (no difference in safety profile)
PROGESTOGENS	• Oral • Intramuscular injection • Intrauterine System (IUS)	Bloating, weight gain, acne, amenorrhoea, mood swings, breast tenderness, irregular bleeding	• *Cochrane Review* concluded that continuous progestogens are effective therapies for treatment of endometriosis-associated pain
GnRH AGONISTS – Also called GnRH **ANALOGUES**	• Intramuscular • Subcutaneous • Intranasal	• Common side effects of agonists are related to decreased oestrogen level and are like the side effects associated with menopause: Hot flushes, headaches, vaginal dryness, decreased libido, depression • Long-term therapy can result in increased risk of osteoporosis and worsening of diabetes	• *Cochrane Review:* GnRH agonist is more effective than placebo (but inferior to levonorgestrel-releasing IUS) in treating endometriosis-associated pain • Use of these drugs is licensed to be used for a maximum of 6 months • Effectiveness is not dependent on mode of administration • Adding add-back HRT reduces menopause-like side effects and prevents osteoporosis
GnRH ANTAGONISTS	• Oral	• Side effects are mostly associated with hypoestrogenic states such as decreased BMD, hot flushes and mood or sleep disturbance • However, their pharmacokinetic profile tends to be less damaging in comparison to GnRH agonists	• Emerging evidence from *RCT* (randomized controlled trials) suggest that GnRH antagonists are more effective for endometriosis-associated pain • Treatment duration should not exceed 24 months
AROMATASE INHIBITORS	• Oral	Side effects are due to low oestrogen levels: loss of libido, vaginal dryness, insomnia, osteoporosis	Reserved for women with endometriosis-associated pain refractory to other medical or surgical treatment
RELUGOLIX-ESTRADIOL-NORETISTERONE ***RELUGOLIX CT***	***Recently approved by NICE on 13 March 2025*** • Once-daily Oral tablet www.nice.org.uk>guidance>ta1057	Depression (discontinue if severe depression) • DEXA scan recommended before starting if risk factors for osteoporosis. • Relugolix CT can be taken up until menopause	Significant improvement in endometriosis-associated pain and well tolerated • Used for symptomatic treatment of endometriosis in women with a history of previous medical or surgical treatment for their endometriosis • Reduces the need for opioid use or repeated surgical treatment

COC = combined oral contraceptive; GnRH = gonadotropin-releasing hormone; HRT = hormone replacement therapy.

The hormonal treatments are generally preferred, as they stop bleeding and reduce ongoing problems such as pain, whereas other treatment modalities only control symptoms. The aim is to suppress ovarian activity, thus preventing cyclical proliferative changes in endometriotic deposits and reducing the symptoms and risk of scarring associated with the inflammatory response (10).

The magnitude of this treatment effect is similar for all treatments, suggesting that little difference exists in their capacity to reduce pain. Furthermore, symptoms return after cessation of treatment and hormone treatments used to manage endometriosis all have side effects. In addition, although the contraceptive properties of the hormones may be welcome if the woman does not wish to become pregnant, they may be unwanted if fertility is desired.

Avoid Hormonal Treatment in Women Who Are Considering Pregnancy

These hormonal therapies include (1,10):

- *Danazol*: A derivative of the male sex hormone testosterone. It inhibits the secretion of GnRH, causing a decrease in the secretion of LH and FSH by the pituitary gland. Therapy is long-term (6–9 months) and is started on the second day of the cycle. The drug has many side effects. These include weight gain, fluid retention, breast reduction, oily skin and acne, hot flashes and decreased voice timbre
- *Combined oral contraceptive pills (COC)* (oestrogen-progesterone preparations): Their action consists of lowering the level of FSH, thus stabilizing the endometrium and reducing pain. These can be taken conventionally, continuously without a break, or in a tricycling regimen (three packs together). If she cannot have oestrogen then the progesterone-only pill (POP) could be used, but it is important to remember that not all women will experience amenorrhoea, so pain may persist
- *Progestogen preparations (POP)*: POP reduce the level of GnRH and thus the levels of FSH, LH and oestrogen. The most common side effects include fluid retention, weight gain, breast tenderness, spotting and irregular bleeding from the genital tract
- *Progestogens-containing intrauterine system (IUS)*: Levonorgestrel (Mirena) and other IUS may provide relief from pain and are also a long-term treatment. The effect is the same as progestogen preparations. Recommended especially for women with severe pain
- *Other forms of progestogens*: Implants (Nexplanon) or injectables (Depo-provera or Sayana Press) can be used

> *If the initial course of hormonal treatment does not manage symptoms, the woman should be referred to a gynaecologist.*

However, none of these treatments eradicates the disease, they are associated with side effects, and endometriosis-related symptoms can sometimes—but not always—reappear after therapy discontinuation.

GONADOTROPHIN-RELEASING HORMONE (GnRH) ANALOGUE INJECTIONS

These are used for the management of numerous gynaecological conditions including:

- Endometriosis
- Uterine fibroids
- Adenomyosis
- Menorrhagia
- Pelvic pain
- Severe premenstrual syndrome

The commonly used injections are Prostap and Zoladex. Both injections are GnRH analogues and drugs are only available in injection form.

Prostap is administered via the intramuscular or subcutaneous route. The medication is a synthetic hormone that is used to reduce the levels of oestrogen in the body. It is also used to treat prostate cancer in men by reducing levels of testosterone.

It affects the release of hormones from the pituitary gland (luteinizing hormone and follicle stimulating hormone). These hormones stimulate the release of oestrogen and progesterone from the ovaries. When the medication is first administered, there is an initial increase in circulating hormones and an initial flare-up response is caused. Patients may notice a flare-up of symptoms associated with their gynaecological condition, but this should only last for the first 2 weeks of treatment.

Ongoing treatment will however cause a reduction of circulating hormones resulting in reduced oestrogen levels, which prevents ovulation and, in turn, causes a medically induced menopause. This menopausal state (anovulation) deprives the endometrial deposits from oestrogen aiming to stop menstrual periods and reduce the associated pelvic pain.

Most women will stop bleeding and notice an improvement to symptoms within 2 months of starting treatment once hormone levels have reduced to a stabilized level.

Side Effects

Most of the side effects are related to decreased oestrogen levels and are similar to the side effects associated with menopause, such as hot flushes, mood swings, depression and vaginal dryness.

GnRH injections may also increase the risk of osteoporosis. Vaginal bleeding may occur during treatment. Blood sugar level may be altered with GnRH analogues.

- *Very common side effects* (may affect more than 1 in 10 people) include difficulty sleeping, headaches or hot flushes
- *Common side effects* (may affect up to 1 in 10 people) include weight changes, mood changes, depression, tingling in hands or feet, dizziness, nausea, joint pain, muscle weakness, breast tenderness, changes in breast size, vaginal dryness and swelling in ankles or skin reactions at the injection site (these include skin hardening, redness, pain, abscesses, swelling)

How Can These Side Effects Be Managed?

As the side effects of GnRH are mainly associated with low oestrogen levels, symptoms can be managed with the use of hormone replacement therapy (HRT).

HRT is usually given alongside GnRH injections to prevent or reduce the side effects associated with menopause making treatment more tolerable.

The most serious side effect of GnRH analogue treatment is thinning of the bones (osteoporosis). Where GnRH analogue treatment is provided for long-term management, a bone density scan [Dual Energy X-ray Absorptiometry (DEXA)] should be carried out after 2 years of treatment to ensure bone density is within the normal range.

Dosage

For both Prostap and Zoladex, there are two doses available:

- Prostap 3.75 mg (4 weekly)
- Prostap 11.25 mg (12 weekly)
- Zoladex 3.6 mg (4 weekly)
- Zoladex 10.8 mg (12 weekly)

> *The dose administered depends on how long the drug is effective. This is decided by the endometriosis specialist consultant.*

AROMATASE INHIBITORS

Letrozole and anastrozole may be prescribed in combination with other hormonal treatment. Their action takes advantage of the fact of specific behaviour of endometriosis cells. Foci of endometriosis, regardless of the ovaries, produce oestrogens that cause an increase in endometrial lesions. Aromatase inhibitors interrupt oestrogen production in both endometriosis foci and ovaries, causing a significant reduction in oestrogen levels.

Side effects are due to low oestrogen levels. The most important of these is the significant loss of calcium from the bones causing osteoporosis. Others include loss of libido, vaginal dryness and insomnia (11).

ELAGOLIX GnRH RECEPTOR ANTAGONIST

The latest drug to be approved by the US Food and Drug Administration (FDA) is Elagolix, for the treatment of moderate to severe pain associated with endometriosis (12). The results of a study in which about 1,700 women with moderate or severe pain in endometriosis participated played a part in the approval. Doses of this drug—150 mg once a day or 200 mg twice a day—significantly reduced the most common types of endometrial pain: pelvic pain and sex-related pain. For a dose of 150 mg, the duration of use of the drug is 24 months; for a dose of 200 mg, duration is limited to 6 months, as the drug causes a decrease in bone mineral density. The drug is taken orally (12).

Elagolix is a non-peptide GnRH (gonadotropin-releasing hormone) antagonist. Elagolix enables dose-dependent reductions in oestrogen levels and is effective in relieving moderate to severe endometriosis pain with long-lasting, sustained effects. As a GnRH antagonist, Elagolix may also reduce bone mineral density through its oestrogen-reduction mechanism (13).

As evidenced by literature data, although there is a risk of bone loss when Elagolix is used, the effect of Elagolix on the long-term risk of fracture is minimal (14,15).

Results from the final model simulations indicate support for recommendations for the use of Elagolix at a dose of 150 mg once daily for 24 months (16).

HORMONAL/MEDICAL THERAPIES FOR ENDOMETRIOSIS-ASSOCIATED INFERTILITY

No evidence exists of benefit of suppression of ovarian function in women with endometriosis-associated infertility who wish to conceive (17). Following surgery for endometriosis, women seeking pregnancy should not be treated with postoperative hormone suppression with the sole purpose of enhancing future pregnancy rates.

Provide Information and Support

The charity Endometriosis UK (18) has many useful online resources for patients, clinicians, family members and carers, as well as clinical education resources. NICE's patient decision aid, *Hormone treatment for endometriosis symptoms—What are my options?* (9) also lists the risks and benefits of the available hormonal treatment options and can be used to empower women to make informed choices about their short- and long-term treatment (9).

It is important that clinicians recognize that the impact of endometriosis goes beyond physical symptoms such as pain and refer patients to support services, for example, for help with anxiety and depression, if indicated.

A sample of a patient information leaflet "GnRH Analogues for Pelvic Pain" can be accessed via www.routledge.com/9781032684796 (made available with permission from Northern Care Alliance NHS Foundation Trust).

Shared Decisions

The Women's Health Strategy published in December 2021 clearly states that women must be involved in decision-making. They should be informed about the evidence and side effects of their chosen form of treatment.

Monitoring of Symptoms

Every patient should be followed up in primary care. Follow-up must include psychological wellbeing in women with confirmed endometriosis.

Regular USS or imaging is not needed unless there is deterioration of symptoms and no benefit with medication.

Follow-up, including psychological support, should be considered in women with confirmed endometriosis, with renewed evaluation and a revised treatment plan if new symptoms emerge, recur or worsen over time.

Given growing evidence of risk of multisystem-involving conditions, monitoring by general practitioners for new emergence of signs and symptoms of mental health conditions, cardiovascular disease, immunologic and autoimmune disorders, gastrointestinal conditions or multifocal pain conditions should be provided and referral to a non-gynaecologic specialist should be considered as needed (19).

KEY POINT SUMMARY

- NICE recommends an initial 3-month trial of paracetamol or non-steroidal anti-inflammatory drugs (NSAIDs) alone or with a combined combined oral contraceptive (COC) pill or continuous progestogen.
- Also offer holistic management for psychological support, fertility priorities, need for contraception and future pregnancy planning.

REFERENCES

1. NICE. *Endometriosis: Diagnosis and management.* NICE Guideline 73. NICE. 2017. www.nice.org.uk/ng73 (accessed 25 Aug 2023).
2. Kalaitzopoulos DR, Samartzis N, Kolovos GN, et al. Treatment of endometriosis: A review with comparison of 8 guidelines. *BMC Womens Health* 2021;21:397. doi:10.1186/s12905-021-01545-5 pmid:34844587 [CrossRef] [PubMed] [Google Scholar]
3. Dunselman G, Vermeulen N, Becker C, et al. ESHRE guideline: Management of women with endometriosis. *Hum Reprod* 2014;29(3):400–12.
4. Endometriosis UK Website. *Pain relief for endometriosis.* www.endometriosis-uk.org/pain-relief-endometriosis (accessed 12 Jan 2023).
5. Kauppila A, Rönnberg L. Naproxen sodium in dysmenorrhea secondary to endometriosis. *Obstet Gynecol* 1985;65:379–83. pmid:3883265 [PubMed] [Web of Science] [Google Scholar]
6. Horne AW, Daniels J, Hummelshoj L, Cox E, Cooper KG. Surgical removal of superficial peritoneal endometriosis for managing women with chronic pelvic pain: Time for a rethink? *BJOG* 2019;126:1414–6. doi:10.1111/1471-0528.15894. [PMC free article] [PubMed] [CrossRef] [Google Scholar]
7. NICE. *Neuropathic pain in adults: Pharmacological management in non-specialist settings.* NICE Clinical Guideline 173. NICE. 2013 (updated Sep 2020). www.nice.org.uk/cg173 (accessed 25 Aug 2023).
8. Horne AW, Vincent K, Hewitt CA, et al. Gabapentin for chronic pelvic pain in women (GaPP2): A multicentre, randomised, double-blind, placebo-controlled trial. *Lancet* 2020;396:909–17. doi:10.1016/S0140-6736(20)31693-7 pmid:32979978
9. Coxon L, Horne AW, Vincent K. Pathophysiology of endometriosis-associated pain: A review of pelvic and central nervous system mechanisms. *Best Pract Res Clin Obstet Gynaecol* 2018;51:53–67. doi:10.1016/j.bpobgyn.2018.01.014 pmid:29525437
10. NICE. *Hormone treatment for endometriosis symptoms—What are my options?* NICE Patient Decision Aid. NICE. 2017. www.nice.org.uk/guidance/ng73/resources/patient-decision-aid-hormone-treatment-for-endometriosis-symptoms-what-are-my-options-pdf-4595573197 (accessed 26 Aug 2023).

11. Donnez J, Dolmans MM. Endometriosis and medical therapy: From progestogens to progesterone resistance to GnRH antagonists: A review. *J Clin Med* 2021;10:1085. doi:10.3390/jcm10051085. [PMC free article] [PubMed] [CrossRef] [Google Scholar]
12. Taylor HS, Giudice LC, Lessey BA, et al. Treatment of endometriosis-associated pain with Elagolix, an oral GnRH antagonist. *N Engl J Med* 2017;377:28–40. doi:10.1056/NEJMoa1700089. [PubMed] [CrossRef] [Google Scholar]
13. Shebley M, Polepally AR, Nader A, et al. Clinical pharmacology of Elagolix: An oral gonadotropin-releasing hormone receptor antagonist for endometriosis. *Clin Pharm* 2020;59:297–309. doi:10.1007/s40262-019-00840-7. [PMC free article] [PubMed] [CrossRef] [Google Scholar]
14. Bradley CA. Reproductive endocrinology: Elagolix in endometriosis. *Nat Rev Endocrinol* 2017;13:439. doi:10.1038/nrendo.2017.74. [PubMed] [CrossRef] [Google Scholar]
15. Kilpatrick RD, Chiuve SE, Leslie WD, et al. Estimating the effect of Elagolix treatment for endometriosis on postmenopausal bone outcomes: A model bridging phase III trials to an older real-world population. *JBMR Plus* 2020;4:e10401. doi:10.1002/jbm4.10401. [PMC free article] [PubMed] [CrossRef] [Google Scholar]
16. Abbas Suleiman A, Nader A, Winzenborg I, et al. Exposure-safety analyses identify predictors of change in bone mineral density and support Elagolix labeling for endometriosis-associated pain: CPT pharmacometrics. *Syst Pharm* 2020;9:639–48. [PMC free article] [PubMed] [Google Scholar]
17. Hughes E, Brown J, Collins JJ, et al. Ovulation suppression for endometriosis. *Cochrane Database Syst Rev* 2007;2007(3):CD000155.
18. Endometriosis UK Website. *Endometriosis UK*. www.endometriosis-uk.org (accessed 25 Sep 2023).
19. Horne AW, Missmer SA. Pathophysiology, diagnosis, and management of endometriosis. *BMJ* 2022;379:e070750. doi:10.1136/bmj-2022-070750 (accessed 20 Aug 2023).

FURTHER READING

European Society of Human Reproduction and Embryology. *Endometriosis: Guideline of European Society of Human Reproduction and embryology.* ESHRE. 2022. www.eshre.eu/Guidelines

NICE. *Hormone treatment for endometriosis symptoms—What are my options?* NICE Patient Decision Aid. NICE. 2017. www.nice.org.uk/guidance/ng73/resources/patient-decision-aid-hormone-treatment-for-endometriosis-symptoms-what-are-my-options-pdf-4595573197 (accessed 25 Aug 2023).

CHAPTER 8

Pelvic Physiotherapy in the Management of Endometriosis

···

Physiotherapy in endometriosis focuses on non-invasive and conservative treatment of pelvic floor disorders in women. It deals with the restoration of the efficiency and function of tissues and organs in the pelvic area, supports the process of surgical treatment, and relieves pain, thus improving the quality of life (QoL) (1). In its various forms, physiotherapy can be an excellent complement to the gynaecological treatment of endometriosis, by virtue of reducing inflammation and alleviating pain, thus significantly improving women's QoL.

Physiotherapy is not included in the NICE Guidelines for endometriosis (2) but is in the NICE Guidelines for chronic pelvic pain (3). It is not a part of care provided to women diagnosed with endometriosis, who are symptomatic, or even before or after surgery in a secondary care setting.

Endometriosis is a systemic disease rather than a disease predominantly affecting the pelvis; therefore, it is important that a holistic approach to management is taken, avoiding an 'end-organ' focus. It is important that sufficient resources and support are prioritized to enable clinicians to continue expanding the current evidence base of physiotherapy treatment to help women with endometriosis. As many of the pain symptoms and co-existing disorders associated with endometriosis are pelvic, pelvic health physiotherapists have a role to play in pain management, with their training in gynaecological, urological and gastroenterological conditions, including pelvic floor dysfunction and persistent pelvic pain.

The use of physiotherapy in women with endometriosis has a complementary effect on the gynaecological, pharmacological and surgical

DOI: 10.1201/9781032684819-8

treatment process. Treatment with physical methods can be an alternative to other forms of treatment. Physiotherapy for patients with endometriosis is a complex therapy and should have a systemic effect (4). An increasing number of women with endometriosis report anecdotal benefit from pelvic physiotherapy.

Physiotherapists may support women with activity management, for example, exercises, pacing strategies and goal setting and/or use complementary approaches to manage their pelvic pain symptoms, for example, massage and trigger point release therapy. Physiotherapists with training in both abdomino-pelvic and general musculoskeletal disorders, as well as persistent pain management, are ideally placed to contribute to the multidisciplinary team approach. A specialist endometriosis centre should have access to a multidisciplinary pain management service with expertise in pelvic pain.

Physiotherapy in endometriosis focuses on different areas of work with patients: preoperative physiotherapy, postoperative physiotherapy, scar therapy and physiotherapy concentrating on pelvic floor work (urogynaecological physiotherapy). Physiotherapy for patients with endometriosis mainly focuses on kinesiotherapy, physical therapy and balneology, as well as the use of manual therapy targeting the lumbo-pelvic area and visceral therapy. Physical activity undertaken by women with endometriosis, learning self-therapy and self-relaxation are also very important.

TYPES OF PHYSIOTHERAPY

Kinesiotherapy

This therapy is based on working with the musculoskeletal system of the reproductive organs and using massage which will include the pelvic area (5). Kinesiotherapy for patients with endometriosis is an important part of treatment and involves the selection of an appropriate exercise programme with individually selected loads. Appropriately selected exercises in the postoperative period and during the treatment of inflammation have a significant effect on the patient's recovery and functioning. Kinesiotherapy is also suitable for patients whose health status rules out surgical treatment.

Physical Therapy

The kinds of physical therapy used in women with endometriosis are mainly light therapy, laser therapy, electrotherapy and magnetotherapy (6–11). Physical therapy treatments complement the comprehensive therapy of endometriosis treatment.

In the field of phototherapy, infrared, red, ultraviolet and visible rays are used. Their main action is to accelerate the absorption of exudates and to improve blood circulation and regeneration after surgery.

Laser Therapy

The use of laser bio-stimulation aims to accelerate tissue healing and regeneration; improve microcirculation in the wound area; and accelerate the growth of fibroblasts, collagen or nerve fibres.

Using low-energy laser radiation, an analgesic and anti-inflammatory effect is also achieved (12).

The use of laser therapy in the treatment of endometriosis is also based on the use of far-infrared low-level laser (light) therapy (LLLT). These treatments have the effect of deeply regenerating and restoring tissue function. Studies show that deep infrared action can increase the proliferation and functional cellular capacity of the endometrium. At the tissue level, there is an acceleration of blood and lymph circulation, a decrease in intracapillary pressure, an increase in the excitability threshold of nerve endings and stimulation of the immune system (13).

Electromagnetic Field

The application of an electromagnetic field generates endogenous (i.e., internal) overheating of the tissues. The treatment is performed on the lower abdominal area. It is used in the treatment of chronic conditions where deep overheating and hyperaemia are indicated. It should not be used in women who are pregnant or trying to get pregnant. In this group of patients, it is advisable to use a pulse wave as a similar effect is obtained with almost complete elimination of the heat factor (14).

Electrotherapy

The physiotherapeutic management of patients with endometriosis also includes electrotherapy, which has an analgesic and hyperaemic effect. Medium and low frequency currents are used (7,8). Both interference currents and transcutaneous electrical nerve stimulation (TENS) have the effect of reducing pain in the pelvic area.

Preoperative Physiotherapy

If surgery is planned, then, prior to the surgery, the patient is taught general conditioning exercises to prevent possible postoperative complications. Rehabilitation begins with breathing exercises and then lower limb exercises are introduced: foot ankle circles, alternating dorsal and sole flexion of the foot. In order to facilitate the outflow of blood and lymph towards the heart, it is advisable to perform these exercises in such a way that the limb is slightly raised above the body.

Postoperative Physiotherapy

Physiotherapy is also provided in the recovery room. Immobilization after surgery can contribute to circulatory disorders and peripheral venous blood retention and increase the risk of thromboembolic and respiratory complications. It is important that the standard of physiotherapy management is for the patient to adopt an upright position as soon as possible and to gradually become mobile, initially at the bedside and then within the patient's room. The point at which the patient may stand upright and at which physiotherapy may be initiated in patients having undergone gynaecological surgery is established according to medical indications and also the individual condition of the patient, her age, existing additional conditions or possible complications following surgery.

If there are no medical contraindications, physiotherapy is started on the first postoperative day. In the case of a laparotomy, the patient changes positions from lying on her back to lying on her side and vice versa, with her lower limbs bent at the hip and knee joints (and thus her abdominal muscles relaxed) by performing a rotation of her entire torso. Once a sitting position is reached, upright positioning is introduced.

Limitations

Two small pilot studies assessed the outcome of manipulations and massage for relief of endometriosis-associated pain specifically, but they included specific patient groups and need expansion and replication to support recommendations for care of endometriosis patients (15,16).

Contraindications for Physiotherapy

Contraindications include:

- Malignant tumours of the reproductive organs prior to 12 months after completion of surgical therapy, radiotherapy or chemotherapy excluding hormonal therapy
- Acute inflammation within the reproductive organs
- Acute bacterial infections or fungal infections

- Established large myomas qualifying for surgical treatment
- Unexplained bleeding from the reproductive tract
- Pregnancy

KEY POINT SUMMARY

- Physiotherapy is safe and effective and can make a significant difference to the symptoms associated with pelvic dysfunction and, therefore, to women's quality of life.
- Pulsed high-intensity laser therapy, transcutaneous electrical nerve stimulation (TENS), pulsed electromagnetic fields and manual physiotherapy are the most effective treatments to reduce pain and improve QoL.
- Despite the positive impact of physiotherapy resulting from its practical use in women with endometriosis, there is a lack of scientific publications of a research nature.
- Establishing the independent benefit of standalone physiotherapy is difficult because most studies have assessed it in combination with psychological and medical management (17).

REFERENCES

1. Vural M. Pelvic pain rehabilitation. *Turk J Phys Med Rehabil* 2018;64:291–9. doi:10.5606/tftrd.2018.3616. [PMC free article] [PubMed] [CrossRef] [Google Scholar]
2. *Endometriosis: Diagnosis and management—NICE*. www.nice.org.uk/guidance/NG73
3. *Overview|Chronic pain (primary and secondary) in over 16s*. www.nice.org.uk/guidance/NG193
4. De Graaff AA, D'Hooghe TM, Dunselman GA, et al. The significant effect of endometriosis on physical, mental and social wellbeing: Results from an international cross-sectional survey. *Hum Reprod* 2013;28:2677–85. doi:10.1093/humrep/det284. [PubMed]
5. Tennfjord MK, Gabrielsen R, Tellum T. Effect of physical activity and exercise on endometriosis-associated symptoms: A systematic review. *BMC Womens Health* 2021;21:355. doi:10.1186/s12905-021-01500-4.] [PubMed]
6. Thabet AAE, Alshehri MA. Effect of pulsed high-intensity laser therapy on pain, adhesions, and quality of life in women having endometriosis: A randomized controlled trial. *Photomed Laser Surg* 2018;36:363–9. doi:10.1089/pho.2017.4419. [PubMed]
7. Mira TAA, Yela DA, Podgaec S, et al. Hormonal treatment isolated versus hormonal treatment associated with electrotherapy for pelvic pain control in deep endometriosis: Randomized clinical trial. *Eur J Obstet Gyneacol Reprod Biol* 2020;255:134–41. doi:10.1016/j.ejogrb.2020.10.018
8. Mira TA, Giraldo PC, Yeala DA, et al. Effectiveness of complementary pain treatment for women with deep endometriosis through transcutaneous

electrical nerve stimulation (TENS): Randomized controlled trial. *Eur J Obstet Gyneacol Reprod Biol* 2015;194:1–6. doi:10.1016/j.ejogrb.2015.07.009

9. Zhang ZY, Wang J, Fan YL, et al. Effectiveness of neuromuscular electrical stimulation for endometriosis-related pain: A protocol of systematic review and meta-analysis. *Medicine* 2020;99:e20483. doi:10.1097/MD.0000000000020483. [PubMed]

10. de Mira TAA, Yela DA, Podgaec S, et al. Reply to letter to the editor entitled "re: Hormonal treatment isolated versus hormonal treatment associated with electrotherapy for pelvic pain control in deep endometriosis: Randomized clinical trial". *Eur J Obstet Gynecol Reprod Biol* 2021;258:463–4. doi:10.1016/j.ejogrb.2021.01.022. [PubMed]

11. Jorgensen WA, Frome BM, Wallach C. Electrochemical therapy of pelvic pain: Effects of pulsed electromagnetic fields (PEMF) on tissue trauma. *Eur J Surg Suppl* 1994;574:83–6. [PubMed]

12. El Faham DA, Elnoury MAH, Morsy MI, et al. Has the time come to include low-level laser photobiomodulation as an adjuvant therapy in the treatment of impaired endometrial receptivity? *Lasers Med Sci* 2018;33:1105–14. doi:10.1007/s10103-018-2476-y. [PubMed]

13. Punnonen R, Grönroos M, Liukko P, et al. The use of pulsed high-frequency therapy (curapuls) in gynecology and obstetrics. *Acta Obstet Gynecol Scand* 1980;59:187–8. doi:10.3109/00016348009154639. [PubMed]

14. Krynicka I, Rutowski R, Staniszewska-Kuś J, et al. The role of laser biostimulation in early post-surgery rehabilitation and its effect on wound healing. *Ortop Traumatol Rehabil* 2010;12:67–79. [PubMed] [Google Scholar]

15. Daraï C, Deboute O, Zacharopoulou C, et al. Impact of osteopathic manipulative therapy on quality of life of patients with deep infiltrating endometriosis with colorectal involvement: Results of a pilot study. *Eur J Obstet Gynecol Reprod Biol* 2015;188:70–3. doi:10.1016/j.ejogrb.2015.03.001 pmid:25796057 [CrossRef] [PubMed] [Google Scholar]

16. Valiani M, Ghasemi N, Bahadoran P, et al. The effects of massage therapy on dysmenorrhea caused by endometriosis. *Iran J Nurs Midwifery Res* 2010;15:167–71. pmid:21589790 [PubMed] [Google Scholar]

17. Loving S, Nordling J, Jaszczak P, et al. Does evidence support physiotherapy management of adult female chronic pelvic pain? A systematic review. *Scand J Pain* 2012;3:70–81. doi:10.1016/j.sjpain.2011.12.002 pmid:29913781 [CrossRef] [PubMed] [Google Scholar]

FURTHER READING

Overview|Chronic pain (primary and secondary) in over 16s. www.nice.org.uk/guidance/NG193

CHAPTER 9

Non-Pharmacological Management

....

The management of endometriosis requires a holistic approach focused on reducing overall inflammation and reducing troublesome symptoms. Improving lifestyle, making changes in the diet, reducing high-fat diet and alcohol consumption can help women with endometriosis to control their disease or at least find symptomatic relief. A dietician may provide great benefit in the management of these patients, especially at younger ages and in early stages.

At present, there is no known way to prevent or cure endometriosis. Enhanced awareness, followed by early diagnosis and management, may slow or halt the natural progression of the disease and reduce the long-term burden of its symptoms, including possibly the risk of central nervous system pain sensitization.

Endometriosis-related symptoms can affect not only woman's physical but also mental and social wellbeing. It causes a significant deterioration in the quality of life (QoL) (1,2). However, the management of these symptoms is not standardized, and the disease can recur even after proper surgical (3) or pharmacological management (4). On the other hand, medical therapy acts with a suppressive effect on endometriosis. Cessation of medical therapy results in reactivation of endometriosis.

Physiotherapists may support women with activity management (for example, exercises, pacing strategies and goal-setting) and/or use complementary approaches to manage their pelvic pain symptoms (for example, massage and trigger point-release therapy).

DOI: 10.1201/9781032684819-9

REGULAR EXERCISE

Regular exercise has a protective effect against inflammatory diseases because it induces an increase in systemic levels of cytokines with anti-inflammatory properties (5).

Regular exercise is thought to promote reduced menstrual flow, ovarian stimulation and oestrogen effects (6).

Analysis of the available literature data shows that there are no controlled and randomized trials determining whether and to what extent exercise can be beneficial for women with endometriosis. So far, researchers have only speculated on this subject (7).

However, there are data that draw attention to the possibility of inferring the non-protective effects of exercise in women with endometriosis, which may result from the discomfort felt that prevents physical exercise (8,9).

Physical exercise has been shown to have a beneficial effect on muscle relaxation in patients suffering from endometriosis, which, in turn, helps to break their pain cycle (8).

Progressive muscle relaxation training has been shown to be more effective in reducing pain, anxiety and depression in women with endometriosis undergoing hormone therapy (10).

Exercise is one of the most effective strategies for increasing serotonin levels; physical activity and deep breathing exercises can increase the rate of burning serotonin neurons in the brain, which can stimulate the production of mood-enhancing substances. Aerobic exercise, such as walking and swimming, can have a more significant effect on serotonin levels, strengthening the muscles of the whole body and improving overall circulation (11).

The relationship between childhood and adolescent weights and the development of endometriosis is counterbalanced. Early studies described the current state of being thin and underweight as hallmarks of patients suffering from endometriosis, without insight into whether this is a cause or a consequence of their disease or its symptoms (12,13).

Regardless of the patient's age, current evidence suggests an inverse relationship between BMI and the prevalence of endometriosis (14). However, the association between obesity and endometriosis remains debatable.

Some researchers have discovered an elevated incidence of endometriosis in obese women with a correlation between the risk of developing endometriosis and prepubertal obesity (15).

Women who reported being overweight at 10 years of age had an increased risk of endometriosis (OR = 2.8; 95% CI: 1.1–7.5), whereas there was no clear evidence of an association between relative weight at 16 years of age and the risk of endometriosis (15,16).

A significant inverse association was found in a meta-analysis This meta-analysis revealed a 33% reduction in the risk of endometriosis for each 5 kg/m^2 increase in BMI (RR = 0.67; 95% CI: 0.53–0.84), with statistically significant heterogeneity across the studies (p < 0.001, I = 86.9%) (17).

PSYCHOLOGICAL AND MENTAL WELLBEING

Endometriosis can cause suffering, distress and economic hardship for individuals and delays in diagnosis can have a significant impact both socially and psychologically (18).

Counselling, CBT therapy and relaxation techniques like yoga, meditation, massage and acupuncture may be beneficial.

Antidepressants and anxiolytics are not the first line of management.

The most common psychologically based intervention for chronic pain is cognitive behavioural therapy (CBT). Most of the studies of CBT in women with endometriosis are of low quality, designed using different methods and based on different psychological frameworks (making separation of effects difficult). However, given that CBT has been evaluated across a spectrum of other chronic pain disorders and shown to be effective for developing pain coping strategies (18,19), it should be integrated into individualized treatment plans when needed.

DIETARY INTERVENTION

Inflammation, oestrogen activity, menstrual regularity and prostaglandin physiology are important pathophysiologic processes to consider when diagnosing and treating endometriosis (20). Diet is an integral component of these factors, and, as such, consumption likely has a role in the development and progression of this disease. In fact, a recent case-control study found that women who consume diets with high inflammatory potential are significantly more likely to have endometriosis in comparison to those with less inflammatory diets (21).

Methylation changes (22), which are a hallmark of cancers and endometriosis (23), are influenced by dietary factors such as folate consumption, calorie intake and polyphenol content. Such compounds tend to bioaccumulate in lipids contained particularly in meat, liver and dairy products and can also be counted among the risk factors for endometrio-sis. However, nowhere in the literature is this association reported.

In a study of curcumin and its impact on endometriosis, the authors found that this spice might have potential benefits for the prevention and treatment of endometriosis. The benefits from curcumin are believed to be due to its anti-inflammatory, antioxidant, anti-tumour and anti-angiogenic profile (24). However, because of the limited studies on this topic and inconsistent data, further studies are needed to improve the knowledge of the true impact of curcumin on endometriosis.

Diet has been postulated to affect symptoms of endometriosis. However, very few studies (all limited quality) have evaluated the ben-efit of dietary interventions and their effect on endometriosis symptoms. Supplements, such as omega-3 polyunsaturated fatty acids (O-PUFAs), have been investigated as a way of reducing inflammation and pain in endometriosis (25,26).

In a recent review, decreased pain scores were observed in women with endometriosis after use of O-PUFAs which were not seen in controls (27). Clinicians should be aware that women with endometriosis have an increased risk of copresenting with irritable bowel syndrome (IBS) con-comitant with endometriosis-associated dyschezia (28). Patients are not uncommonly referred to gastroenterology evaluation without considera-tion of potential endometriosis (29).

High-Fat Diet

High-fat consumption is associated with oxidative stress and inflammation—two key features of endometriosis. Some inflammatory markers, such as interleukin-6 (IL-6), are found in higher concentrations in women with endometriosis and are increased by specific fatty acid exposure (30). Heard et al. reported an increase in endometriosis lesion development in mouse models after exposure to a high-fat diet independ-ent of overt obesity and weight gain (31) believed to be due to promoted oxidative stress and inflammatory pathways provoked by high-fat diets. Maintaining a healthy diet has considerable health benefits and may also decrease the risk of endometriosis (31).

Gluten-Free Diet

Evidence seen of a woman suffering from endometriosis with concomi-tant coeliac disease, where a gluten-free diet improved her fertility (32). The gluten-free diet was tested in 207 symptomatic women suffering from endometriosis, and this reported a statistically significant improvement in symptoms in 75% of the women (33). Women exposed to a gluten-free diet had a significantly better quality of life in addition to improved physical and social functioning ($p < 0.005$) (32). Both endometriosis and coeliac disease are associated with chronic inflammation, and both present with significant elevations of interferon-gamma (IFN-γ) and interleukin-6 (IL-6). Thus, the authors concluded that a gluten-free diet is efficient in improving endometriosis symptoms after 12 months of treatment and plays an antagonist role by decreasing IFN-γ and IL-6 (33).

Fasting

Fasting can help preserve energy levels, thereby providing the body time to regenerate and heal. Increased hormonal modulation and reduced inflammation (34) are ways in which fasting may help reduce chronic pain severity. Currently, there are no studies on the role of fasting in the management of endometriosis.

Alcohol

Studies have shown that drinking too much alcohol can raise the amount of oestrogen the body makes, which could lead to endometriosis. General advice is to stick to no more than one alcohol drink per day.

Data are mixed regarding alcohol consumption and the development of endometriosis (35–37). Several studies have identified an association between alcohol consumption and symptoms related to endometriosis, whereas others have not (36,38). Still, the available evidence is not without limitations. In the studies where researchers found an association between endometriosis and alcohol consumption, it is difficult to ascertain whether the consumption is due to the disease or vice versa. Currently, it also remains unknown whether different types of alcohol affect this disease differently.

Caffeine

Amongst others, caffeine has been studied extensively during the last decade as a putative contributing factor.

Caffeine consumption does not appear to be associated with increased risk for endometriosis. However, further research is needed to elucidate the potential dose-dependent link between caffeine and endometriosis or the probable role of caffeine intake as a measurement of other unidentified biases (40).

BREASTFEEDING

Among women who experienced at least one pregnancy that lasted at least 6 months, breastfeeding was inversely associated with risk of incident endometriosis. This association was partially influenced by postpartum amenorrhea, suggesting that breastfeeding could influence the risk of endometriosis both through amenorrhea and other mechanisms. Given the chronic and incurable nature of endometriosis, breastfeeding should be further investigated as an important modifiable behaviour to mitigate risk for pregnant women (39).

KEY POINT SUMMARY

- Despite the low level of evidence, there are frequent associations between endometriosis and GI conditions in addition to the influence of different nutritional factors on the disease.
- There is also evidence that the adaptation of individualized dietary changes yields statistically significant improvements in endometriosis-related symptoms (41).
- Thus, there may be great benefit to including a dietician in the management of these patients, especially at younger ages and in early stages.
- Counselling, CBT therapy and relaxation techniques like yoga, meditation, massage and acupuncture may be beneficial.
- The management of endometriosis requires a holistic approach focused on reducing overall inflammation, increasing detoxification and attenuating troublesome symptoms. Inarguably, further research with a more extensive focus is needed.

REFERENCES

1. Vessey MP, Villerd-Mackintosh L, Painter R. Epidemiology of endometriosis in women attending family planning clinics. *BMJ* 1993;306:182–4. doi:10.1136/bmj.306.6871.182. [PubMed]
2. Vigano P, Parazzini F, Somigliana E, et al. Endometriosis: Epidemiology and eathiological factors. *Best Pract Res Clin Obstet Gynaecol* 2004;18:177–200. doi:10.1016/j.bpobgyn.2004.01.007. [PubMed]
3. D'Alterio MN, Saponara S, D'Ancona G, et al. Role of surgical treatment in endometriosis. *Minerva Obstet Gynecol* 2021;73:317–32. [PubMed]
4. Laganà AS, La Rosa VL. Multidisciplinary management of endometriosis: Current strategies and future challenges. *Minerva Med* 2020;111:18–20. [PubMed]
5. Febbraio MA. Exercise and inflammation. *J Appl Physiol* 2007;103:376–7. doi:10.1152/japplphysiol.00414.2007. [PubMed]
6. Warren MP, Perlroth NE. The effects of intense exercise on the female reproductive system. *J Endocrinol* 2001;170:3–11. doi:10.1677/joe.0.1700003. [PubMed]

7. Koppan A, Hamori J, Vranics I, et al. Pelvic pain in endometriosis: Painkillers or sport to alleviate symptoms? *Acta Physiol Hung* 2010;97:234–9. doi:10.1556/APhysiol.97.2010.2.10. [PubMed]
8. Awad E, Ahmed H, Yousef A, et al. Efficacy of exercise on pelvic pain and posture associated with endometriosis: Within subject design. *J Phys Sci* 2017;29:2112–5. doi:10.1589/jpts.29.2112. [PubMed]
9. Lund I, Lundeberg T. Is acupuncture effective in the treatment of pain in endometriosis? *J Pain Res* 2016;9:157–65. doi:10.2147/JPR.S55580. [PubMed]
10. Zhao L, Wu H, Zhou X, et al. Effects of progressive muscular relaxation training on anxiety, depression, and quality of life of endometriosis patients under gonadotrophin-releasing hormone agonist therapy. *Eur J Obstet Gynecol Reprod Biol* 2012;162:211–5. doi:10.1016/j.ejogrb.2012.02.029. [PubMed]
11. Carpenter SE, Tjaden B, Rock JA, et al. The effect of regular exercise on women receiving danazol for treatment of endometriosis. *Int J Gynaecol Obstet* 1995;49:299–304. doi:10.1016/0020-7292(95)02359-K. [PubMed]
12. McCann SE, Freudenheim JL, Darrow SL, et al. Endometriosis and body fat distribution. *Obstet Gynecol* 1993;82:545–9. [PubMed]
13. Hemmings R, Rivard M, Olive DL, et al. Evaluation of risk factors associated with endometriosis. *Fertil Steril* 2004;81:1513–21. [PubMed]
14. Aarestrup J, Jensen BW, Ulrich LG, et al. Birth weight, childhood body mass index and height and risks of endometriosis and adenomyosis. *Ann Hum Biol* 2020;47:173–80. [PubMed]
15. Nagle CM, Bell TA, Purdie DM, et al. Relative weight at ages 10 and 16 years and risk of endometriosis: A case-control analysis. *Hum Reprod Oxf Engl* 2009;24:1501–6. [PubMed]
16. Holdsworth-Carson SJ, Dior UP, Colgrave EM, et al. The association of body mass index with endometriosis and disease severity in women with pain. *J Endometr Pelvic Pain Disord* 2018;10:79–87.
17. Liu Y, Zhang W. Association between body mass index and endometriosis risk: A meta-analysis. *Oncotarget* 2017;8:46928–36. [PubMed]
18. Culley L, Law C, Hudson N, et al. The social and psychological impact of endometriosis on women's lives: A critical narrative review. *Hum Reprod Update* 2013;19(6):625–39.
19. Cohen SP, Vase L, Hooten WM. Chronic pain: An update on burden, best practices, and new advances. *Lancet* 2021;397:2082–97. doi:10.1016/S0140-6736(21)00393-7 pmid:34062143
20. Jurkiewicz-Przondziono J, Lemm M, Kwiatkowska-Pamuła A, et al. Influence of diet on the risk of developing endometriosis. *Ginekol Pol* 2017;88:96–102. [PubMed]
21. Demézio da Silva CV, Felipe VL, Shivappa N, et al. Dietary inflammatory index score and risk of developing endometriosis: A case-control study. *J Endometr Pelvic Pain Disord* 2021;13:32–9.
22. Maniglio P, Ricciardi E, Laganà AS, et al. Epigenetic modifications of primordial reproductive tract: A common etiologic pathway for Mayer-Rokitansky-Kuster-Hauser syndrome and endometriosis? *Med Hypotheses* 2016;90:4–5. [PubMed]
23. Terzic M, Aimagambetova G, Kunz J, et al. Molecular basis of endometriosis and endometrial cancer: Current knowledge and future perspectives. *Int J Mol Sci* 2021;22:9274. [PubMed]
24. Wu CY, Chang WP, Chang YH, et al. The risk of irritable bowel syndrome in patients with endometriosis during a 5-year follow-up: A nationwide

population-based cohort study. *Int J Colorectal Dis* 2015;30:907–12. [PubMed]

25. Abokhrais IM, Denison FC, Whitaker LHR, et al. A two-arm parallel double-blind randomised controlled pilot trial of the efficacy of Omega-3 polyunsaturated fatty acids for the treatment of women with endometriosis-associated pain (PurFECT1). *PLoS One* 2020;15:e0227695. doi:10.1371/journal.pone.0227695

26. Nodler JL, DiVasta AD, Vitonis AF, et al. Supplementation with vitamin D or ω-3 fatty acids in adolescent girls and young women with endometriosis (SAGE): A double-blind, randomized, placebocontrolled trial. *Am J Clin Nutr* 2020;112:229–36. doi:10.1093/ajcn/nqaa096

27. Huijs E, Nap A. The effects of nutrients on symptoms in women with endometriosis: A systematic review. *Reprod Biomed Online* 2020;41:317–28. doi:10.1016/j.rbmo.2020.04.014

28. DiVasta AD, Zimmerman LA, Vitonis AF, et al. Overlap between irritable bowel syndrome diagnosis and endometriosis in adolescents. *Clin Gastroenterol Hepatol* 2021;19:528–37.e1. doi:10.1016/j.cgh.2020.03.014

29. Singh SS, Missmer SA, Tu FF. Endometriosis and pelvic pain for the gastroenterologist. *Gastroenterol Clin North Am* 2022;51:195–211. doi:10.1016/j.gtc.2021.10.012

30. Bedaiwy MA, Falcone T, Sharma RK, et al. Prediction of endometriosis with serum and peritoneal fluid markers: A prospective controlled trial. *Hum Reprod Oxf Engl* 2002; 7:426–31. [PubMed] [Google Scholar]

31. Heard ME, Melnyk SB, Simmen FA, et al. High-fat diet promotion of endometriosis in an immunocompetent mouse model is associated with altered peripheral and ectopic lesion redox and inflammatory status. *Endocrinology* 2016;157:2870–82. [PubMed] [Google Scholar]

32. Caserta D, Matteucci E, Ralli E, et al. Celiac disease and endometriosis: An insidious and worrisome association hard to diagnose: A case report. *Clin Exp Obstet Gynecol* 2014;41:346–8. [PubMed] [Google Scholar]

33. Marziali M, Venza M, Lazzaro S, et al. Gluten-free diet: A new strategy for management of painful endometriosis related symptoms? *Minerva Chir* 2012;67:499–504. [PubMed] [Google Scholar]

34. Sturlese E, Salmeri FM, Retto G, et al. Dysregulation of the Fas/FasL system in mononuclear cells recovered from peritoneal fluid of women with endometriosis. *J Reprod Immunol* 2011;92:74–81. [PubMed] [Google Scholar]

35. Hemmert R, Schliep KC, Willis S, et al. Modifiable lifestyle factors and risk for incident endometriosis. *Paediatr Perinat Epidemiol* 2019;33:19–25. [PubMed] [Google Scholar]

36. Parazzini F, Esposito G, Tozzi L, et al. Epidemiology of endometriosis and its comorbidities. *Eur J Obstet Gynecol Reprod Biol* 2017;209:3–7. [PubMed] [Google Scholar]

37. Jurkiewicz-Przondziono J, Lemm M, Kwiatkowska-Pamuła A, et al. Influence of diet on the risk of developing endometriosis. *Ginekol Pol* 2017;88:96–102. [PubMed] [Google Scholar]

38. Trabert B, Peters U, De Roos AJ, et al. Diet and risk of endometriosis in a population-based case-control study. *Br J Nutr* 2011;105:459–67. [PubMed]

39. Farland LV, Heather Eliassen A, Tamimi RM. History of breast feeding and risk of incident endometriosis: Prospective cohort study. *BMJ* 2017 Aug 29;358:j3778.

40. Kechagias KS, Triantafyllidis KK, Kyriakidou M, et al. The relation between caffeine consumption and endometriosis: An updated systematic review and mata-analysis. *Nutrients* 2021 Oct 6;13(10).

41. Karlsson JV, Patel H, Premberg A. Experiences of health after dietary changes in endometriosis: A qualitative review study. *BMJ Open* 2020;10:e032321. [PubMed]

FURTHER READING

The Role of Dietary Fats in the Development and Treatment of Endometriosis. Published online 2023 Feb 27. doi:10.3390/life13030654.

CHAPTER 10

Surgical Management: Introduction

....

The book has two chapters on surgical management.

Chapter 10A is contributed by Miss Gaity Ahmad and her two registrars. Miss Ahmad is Clinical Director for Gynaecology, Clinical Lead for the NCA Endometriosis Centre, Honorary Senior Lecturer, Manchester University working in Royal Oldham Hospital and Rochdale Infirmary. She plays a big part in our local Endometriosis Awareness North charity and does regular presentations for local GPs on endometriosis about service provision in a tertiary centre, what is endometriosis surgery, different types of surgery, who needs the surgery and what happens after the surgery including risks and complications. It is important for local GPs to know who to send the referral to, choosing the right consultant to avoid unnecessary delay.

This chapter focuses on surgical management of endometriosis-associated pain: surgery for superficial peritoneal endometriosis, ovarian and deep endometriosis.

The chapter also mentions an increasing interest since the emergence of robot assisted laparoscopy (RAL), but a lack of RCT and no overall evidence to support either RAL or conventional laparoscopy regarding complication rates. More studies are needed for long-term outcomes such as improved quality of life, symptom relief and improved fertility with RAL.

Pre- and postoperative hormonal treatment and recurrence after the surgery with references for detailed information are also included in this chapter.

DOI: 10.1201/9781032684819-10

Chapter 10B is contributed by Professor Andrew Horne, Professor of Gynaecology and Reproductive Sciences, Centre for Reproductive Health, Institute for Regeneration and Repair, University of Edinburgh and Specialty Trainee Obstetrics and Gynaecology and MD Candidate, Centre for Biomedicine.

Professor Horne is the current Chair of the Academic Board at the RCOG, Past Chair of the ESHRE Special Interest Group for Endometriosis and Endometrial Disorders, UK ESHRE National Representative, Trustee/Medical Advisor for the Ectopic Pregnancy Trust, and Trustee/Medical Advisor for Endometriosis UK and the Pelvic Pain Support Network. Persistent pelvic pain and endometriosis are among his research interests. He is currently investigating the aetiology and researching novel treatment approaches of these common clinical problems. Published in *BMJ* in 2022, an article on pathophysiology, diagnosis and management of endometriosis aimed for gynaecologists, GPs and clinicians specializing in conditions for which patients with endometriosis are at higher risk is well written and well-researched and provides valuable and accurate information to the readers that is easy to understand.

He contributed towards developing the Edinburgh Endometriosis Centre of Expertise and is working closely with Endometriosis UK (medical advisor) and the Scottish Parliament to campaign for better care in Scotland for women with endometriosis.

This chapter examines evidence supporting different surgical treatments including surgical management if fertility is a priority, surgery for recurrent symptoms and secondary prevention.

The author mentions hysterectomy as a treatment option for some women, particularly those who have co-existing adenomyosis and those who have exhausted all other treatment options.

CHAPTER 10A

Surgical Management I

....

Shatha Al-Attili, Jamel Tahar Aissa and Gaity Ahmad

Surgical treatment is an important part in the management of endometriosis. The goal of surgery is to eliminate all visible endometriotic peritoneal lesions, endometriomas and deep endometriosis and to divide the associated adhesions aiming to restore normal anatomy of the pelvis.

However, success in reducing pain and increasing pregnancy rates is often dependent on the extent of disease. In addition, lesions may recur even after successful eradication, and pelvic floor muscle abnormalities can contribute to chronic pelvic pain. Secondary changes of the pelvis, including the pelvic floor, and central sensitization may benefit from physiotherapy and complementary treatments.

When surgery is chosen as the treatment option, a laparoscopic approach should be used rather than laparotomy as it carries less pain and morbidity and has a quicker recovery, shorter hospital stay and lower cost on the health care system (1). In addition to that, laparoscopy allows for better visualization of endometriotic lesions. If local expertise is lacking, patients should be referred to a specialized centre where expertise is available and care can be provided in the context of a multidisciplinary team (2).

WHO CAN PERFORM THE SURGICAL TREATMENT?

General Gynaecology Services

Patients with suspected endometriosis and those with severe, persistent and recurrent symptoms that have failed to resolve with initial management (trial of analgesia or hormonal treatment) should be referred

DOI: 10.1201/9781032684819-11

for assessment within the general gynaecology service. The patient will have a detailed history and examination performed in addition to other investigations, which may include a pelvic ultrasound scan or MRI scan. If endometriosis (not involving the bladder, bowel or ureter) is still suspected or diagnosed, then a diagnostic laparoscopy might be considered (2). It should be noted that normal imaging does not exclude the diagnosis. A general gynaecologist should have the training and skills in laparoscopy to be able to do systematic inspection of pelvis, take biopsy for histologic confirmation of diagnosis and treat all visible peritoneal lesions and uncomplicated endometrioma (2).

Endometriosis Specialized Centres and the Endometriosis Multidisciplinary Team (MDT)

However, if the general gynaecologist suspects or has confirmed deep endometriosis (stage III/IV), or the patient is aged 17 and under, a referral should be done to a specialized endometriosis centre (2). The British Society of Gyneacological Endoscopy (BSGE) Subcommittee has worked to establish a network of specialist endometriosis centres to enable patients with severe endometriosis to have access to specialists in the field (3). When performed in specialized centres, laparoscopic excision of rectovaginal disease is effective in treating pain and bowel symptoms with a low rate of major complications (4). A BSGE-accredited endometriosis centre needs to fulfill certain criteria including working in multidisciplinary teams (MDT), recording and auditing outcomes and having a sufficient workload to maintain and develop surgical skills (5).

A specialized endometriosis centre should have access to a multidisciplinary team including the following professionals (2):

- Gynaecologists with expertise in diagnosing and managing endometriosis including advanced laparoscopic surgical skills
- Colorectal surgeon and urologist with interest in endometriosis
- Endometriosis specialist nurse
- Multidisciplinary pain management service
- Health care professional with special interest in gynaecological imaging of endometriosis
- Advanced diagnostic facilities (radiology, histopathology)
- Fertility specialist

Due to the chronicity and complexity of severe endometriosis (physically, mentally and socially for the patient and surgically), there is a need for a combined holistic input of these professionals. Through MDT meetings, there can be more consistent, evidence-based and cost-effective care provided (6). Relevant history, patient preferences, examinations and imaging are all reviewed to localize and assess the extent of disease and operative planning and discuss complication risks. Following this, a consensus recommendation is made and discussed with the patient to decide on further management. Despite the trend and theoretical benefits of an endometriosis MDT, further studies are needed to truly determine the extent of improvements to quality of life when care is provided as an MDT (7).

It is important to discuss patient-specific risks as well as the local unit complication rates with the patients to allow informed decision-making. There are risks of significant complications including the need for a colostomy in case of a bowel injury or planned enterotomy. Patients need to be thoroughly counselled regarding significant risks and complications so they can decide if that is acceptable for them, how this might affect their life and, accordingly, how radical the approach can be in removing the endometriotic tissue.

ROBOTIC COMPARED TO CONVENTIONAL SURGICAL TREATMENT

Since the emergence of robot-assisted laparoscopy (RAL), there has been an interest in its application and using its benefits within the surgically challenging operative management of endometriosis. RAL offers ergonomic and articulating instruments with tremor filtration, which allows for a more precise tissue dissection in addition to three-dimensional, high-definition views of the operative field (8). In theory, this should allow for a more radical excision of diseased tissue.

However, since its emergence, there has been a lack of randomized controlled trials, and there is overall no evidence to support either RAL or conventional laparoscopy regarding complication rates (9–12). One prospective cohort study has shown that RAL may be better than conventional laparoscopy in discoid and segmental resections with lower intraoperative complications and higher rates of healthy tissue margins (13). RAL appears to be associated with longer operating times (10) (due to setting the system up and troubleshooting if there are issues), it is costly compared to other surgical methods (14), and there is a loss of tactile feedback between the tissues and instruments (14). There is only one trial that has looked at 6-month postoperative quality of life outcomes with no significant difference between RAL and conventional laparoscopy (10). There is a lack of studies looking at long-term outcomes (symptom relief, improved fertility and improved quality of life).

INDICATIONS FOR SURGICAL TREATMENT

Surgical treatment for endometriosis may be indicated in the following situations:

1) Refractory symptoms despite analgesic and/or hormonal treatment
2) Fertility improvement

Decision for surgery should be part of shared decision-making between the patient and clinicians taking into account the patient's symptoms, fertility wishes, preferences, previous treatment attempts and patient-specific medico-surgical history. A detailed discussion of surgical management options with patient needs to be done and include talking about:

- What a laparoscopy involves and what surgical treatment can be done
- How laparoscopic surgery could affect her symptoms
- The possible benefits and risks of surgery
- The possible need for further surgery if complications happen
- The possible need for further planned surgery for deep endometriosis involving the bowel, bladder or ureter

SURGICAL TREATMENT FOR PAIN SYMPTOMS

Peritoneal Endometriosis

A *Cochrane Review* concluded that laparoscopic surgery results in improved pain outcome, by reducing overall pain at 6 months, compared to diagnostic surgery alone (15). When comparing immediate excision of peritoneal endometriosis to a two-step approach (diagnostic laparoscopy alone initially, followed by a repeat laparoscopic excision), it was found that a significantly greater number of women in the immediate excision group reported overall pain improvement at 6 months (16). This highlights the importance of a see-and-treat approach when operating. Examples of endometriosis lesions can be seen in Figure 10A.1.

The available methods to eliminate endometriosis lesions include excision and ablation. Ablation can be either by coagulation using diathermy or by CO_2 laser vaporization (1). One meta-analysis showed that excision is significantly superior to ablation in reducing chronic pelvic pain (17),

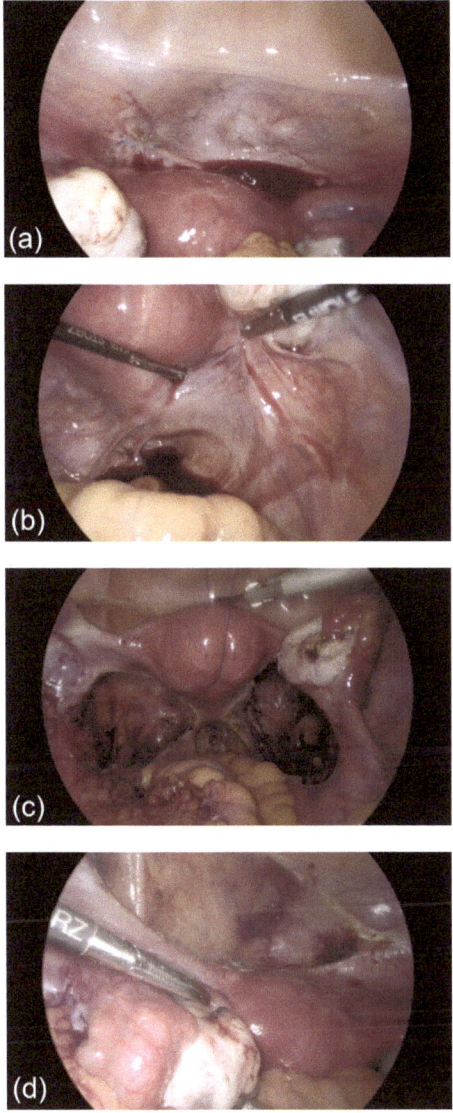

FIGURE 10A.1 Laparoscopic views of pelvis from umbilical port in a patient suffering from dysmenorrhea. (a) Endometriotic lesions located in the uterovesical peritoneal fold. (b) Endometriotic lesion noted in the right pelvic side wall with similar lesions on the left side. (c and d) Views at the end of the procedure where the uterus has been suspended to the abdominal wall during the operation to allow visualization, both pelvic side walls have been excised following identification and mobilization of the ureters, and the uterovesical fold has been excised.

but another recent systematic review showed that there is no difference between ablation and excision in improving symptoms of dysmenorrhea, dyspareunia and dyschezia (18). There is a weak recommendation by the ESHRE guidelines 2022 to consider excision rather than ablation of endometriosis to reduce endometriosis-associated pain. The excisional approach is likely to be more suitable for deep endometriosis lesions, as it is impossible to know if the entire lesion is destroyed with ablative techniques (1).

The effectiveness of surgical interruption of pelvic nerve pathways to control endometriosis-associated pain has been concluded in a Cochrane review that laparoscopic uterosacral nerve ablation (LUNA) did not offer any additional benefit as an adjunct to conservative surgery after 1 year (19). Presacral neurectomy (PSN) performed as an adjunct to laparoscopic surgery for endometriosis is beneficial in the treatment of endometriosis-associated midline pain. However, it requires an advanced level of surgical skills and increases the risk of adverse outcomes such as intraoperative bleeding, postoperative constipation, urinary urgency and painless first stage of labor (19).

After laparoscopic treatment of endometriosis, any hormonal treatment within 6 months can be considered to prolong the benefit of surgery and manage symptoms, if not wishing for immediate conception (1,2).

Ovarian Endometriosis (Endometrioma)

When surgery is performed for endometrioma, it is recommended to do cystectomy (excision of cyst wall) rather than drainage and coagulation using bipolar diathermy (destruction of the inner surface of the cyst wall leaving the cyst in situ), as cystectomy provides a lower recurrence rate and reduces endometriosis-associated pain (20). Ablation treatment using CO_2 laser vaporization can be considered to preserve healthy ovarian tissue. There is a higher recurrence rate with laser vaporization compared to cystectomy within the first year, but the recurrence is similar beyond the first year after surgery (21).

It is important to keep in mind that ovarian surgery has an impact on ovarian reserve and can affect fertility chances and risk of premature menopause. Therefore, caution should be used to minimize ovarian tissue damage. Recent systematic review and meta-analysis confirmed that cystectomy, particularly for bilateral endometriomas, has a deleterious and sustained effect on ovarian reserve (22). Surgery for recurrent endometriomas is more harmful to healthy ovarian tissue and ovarian reserve than the first surgery as demonstrated by removal of larger portions of ovarian tissue (23). The risk of ovarian failure after bilateral ovarian endometrioma removal is reported to be 2.4% (24).

Deep-Infiltrating Endometriosis

Deep endometriosis extends beneath the peritoneum more than 5 mm. Deep endometriosis is more commonly seen in the posterior compartment of the pelvis (uterosacral ligaments, pelvic side walls, rectovaginal septum and bowel), with colorectal involvement reported in 5–12% of women affected by endometriosis (25). In the case of bowel wall infiltration, about 90% is localized in the sigmoid colon or rectum (25). Please see Figure 10A.2 for an example of deep-infiltrating endometriosis.

If there is clinical evidence of deep endometriosis involving the ureter, bladder and bowel, careful consideration should be made as to how to manage this. There is overall a lack of evidence to favor medical or surgical management in cases of deep endometriosis with a similar satisfactory rate of around 70–80% in both groups (26). As mentioned earlier, patients should be referred to a specialized endometriosis centre for investigations and decision-making in an MDT context. The surgery needs to be done as safely as possible and by appropriately trained surgeons with possible involvement of surgeons from other specialties.

Preoperative assessment is important to predict the severity of disease, the difficulty expected and which specialties need to be available, aiming to avoid unnecessary complications and leaving any disease behind. In addition to that, patients should be counselled in detail about what surgery includes and about possible benefits, risks and complications.

Preoperative workup can include MRI to assess the extent of deep endometriosis involving bowel, bladder and ureters. A CT-urogram can detect ureteric stricture and hydronephrosis. A contrast enema or a sigmoidoscopy can detect any narrowing or visible endometriosis lesions at the level of rectum and sigmoid. Perioperative preparations include ureteric stenting if there is hydronephrosis or bladder nodule close to the ureter and bowel preparation.

In general, when surgical treatment for deep endometriosis is chosen, excision of these nodules is usually performed rather than ablation to ensure that the entire lesion is eliminated. As an adjunct to surgery of deep endometriosis, the clinician can consider 3 months of GnRH therapy before surgery to down-regulate the disease (2).

Treatment approaches for colorectal endometriosis include superficial shaving, discoid resection and segmental resection of the bowel to remove the deep larger endometriosis nodules (1). Treatment should be

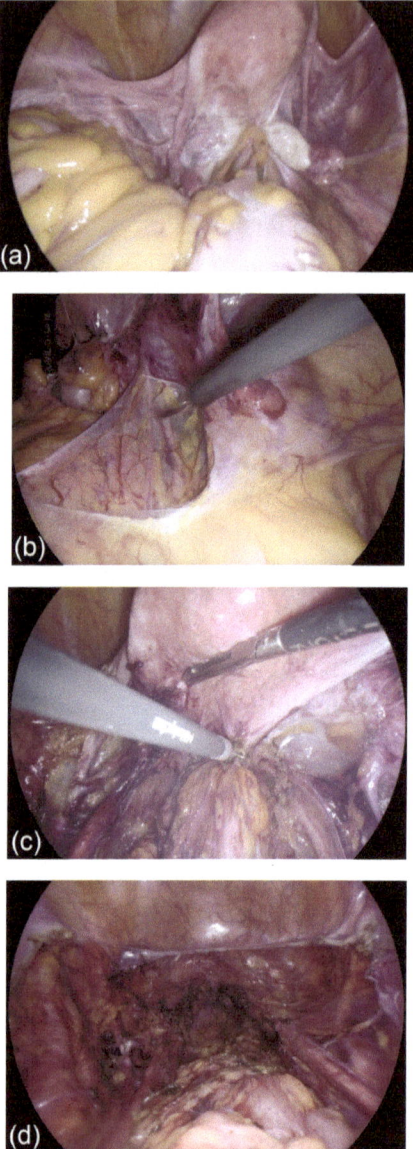

FIGURE 10A.2 Laparoscopic views of pelvis from umbilical port in a patient suffering from dysmenorrhea, menorrhagia and pelvic pain. (a) Both ovaries are adherent to the posterior uterine surface with the sigmoid colon adherent and pinched in between them. (b) Careful ureterolysis where the ureter is clearly identified and freed from the surrounding tissues. This allows for safe excision of the pelvic sidewall, which may contain diseased tissue and allows safer treatment of the bowel endometriosis. (c) Careful release of the bowel from the posterior uterus, in this case with a monopolar hook. Rectal nodule was later shaved off using the same instrument. (d) Views at the end of the procedure following total hysterectomy, bilateral salpingo-oophorecomty and treatment of rectovaginal endometriosis.

done in a multidisciplinary setting with a minimally invasive approach, aiming to remove all endometriosis lesions but also taking into consideration the long-term morbidity of potential complications and respecting the patient's pre-stated wishes regarding how radical the surgical approach should be.

Surgical treatment of bladder endometriosis is usually excision of the lesion and primary closure of the bladder wall. Ureteral lesions may be excised after stenting the ureter; however, in the presence of intrinsic lesions or significant obstruction, segmental excision with end-to-end anastomosis or reimplantation may be necessary (1). Ureterolysis, where the ureter is freed from the surrounding tissue (adhesion or endometriosis) is a conservative approach and is appropriate in most patients with ureteral endometriosis (1).

The largest multicentre prospective case series to date published (4) and the ESHRE Endometriosis Guidelines 2022 (1) suggest a significant reduction in endometriosis-associated pain symptoms, GI and urinary symptoms and improvement in quality of life in surgical management of deep endometriosis. Still, the literature regarding treatment and outcome of deep endometriosis surgery should be interpreted with caution due to the overall low evidence level and lack of randomized controlled trials (1).

Hysterectomy for Endometriosis-Associated Pain

There are no RCTs on hysterectomy for endometriosis-associated pain, but there is a weak recommendation that hysterectomy for endometriosis-associated pain can be effective for relieving symptoms (27,28) and can significantly reduce the need for re-operation (29). Hysterectomy (with or without oophorectomy) with removal of all visible endometriosis lesions should be reserved for women who no longer wish to conceive and who have not responded to more conservative management. Nevertheless, patients should be counselled that hysterectomy will not necessarily cure their symptoms and that it is best reserved for women with coexisting adenomyosis or for women with severe pain who have exhausted all other options to improve their symptoms (30).

The removal of both ovaries will lead to regression of any remaining endometriosis and reduces chances of recurrence, but this will create a state of early menopause and the potential need for HRT. The long-term significance of this depends on the patient's age.

Recent longitudinal studies have not found a benefit of bilateral oophorectomy for long-term pain management (30,31).

Black, indigenous and people of color (BIPOC) women are more likely to have complications of hysterectomy, in part, because they are more likely to undergo laparotomy rather than minimally invasive laparoscopy (32). Women should be informed that hysterectomy is associated with long-term morbidity (33), including cardiovascular disease (34), among those with and without surgically induced menopause (35).

However, it is not a valid option for patients seeking fertility.

RECURRENCE OR PROGRESSION OF ENDOMETRIOSIS AFTER SURGERY

The reported recurrence rate of painful symptoms attributed to endometriosis is high, estimated as 21.5% at 2 years and 40–50% at 5 years (31).

In prospective studies of repeat surgeries, lesions progressed (in 29% of cases), regressed (in 42%), or were static (in 29%) (36). Surgical treatment of certain subtypes of endometriosis could also exacerbate painful symptoms (37).

PRE- AND POSTOPERATIVE HORMONE TREATMENT

Preoperative hormone treatment has not been shown to improve the immediate outcome of surgery for pain, or reduce recurrence, in women with endometriosis (38).

Women with endometriosis who undergo hysterectomy with oophorectomy should be advised to start continuous combined hormone replacement therapy (HRT) for at least the first few years after surgery (39). This may be changed later to oestrogen alone, but this needs to be balanced with the theoretical risk of reactivation and malignant transformation of any residual endometriosis, which can occur many years later.

KEY POINT SUMMARY

- Surgical treatment can be offered as one of the options to treat endometriosis-associated symptoms, especially in cases that fail to respond to medical treatment.
- A shared decision-making approach should be followed based on a woman's symptoms, preferences and priorities.
- Laparoscopy should be the mode of surgery, and well-trained experts should be available to perform surgery.

- In cases of deep endometriosis or recurrent endometriosis, referral to a specialized endometriosis centre should take place and management should be in the context of a multidisciplinary team approach.
- It is recommended to offer surgical treatment for endometriosis-associated pain, as it reduces the pain symptoms.
- There is not enough evidence on the benefit of surgical treatment for endometriosis-associated infertility.

REFERENCES

1. ESHRE. *Endometriosis by the European Society of Human Reproduction and Embryology.* ESHRE. [Online]. www.eshre.eu/Guideline/Endometriosis (accessed 22 Nov 2023).
2. NICE. *Endometriosis: Diagnosis and management.* [Online]. www.nice.org.uk/guidance/ng73 (accessed 22 Nov 2023).
3. BSGE. *Endometriosis centres subcommittee.* [Online]. www.bsge.org.uk/committees/endometriosis-centres/ (accessed 11 Oct 2023).
4. Byrne D, Curnow T, Smith P, et al. Laparoscopic excision of deep rectovaginal endometriosis in BSGE endometriosis centres: A multicentre prospective cohort study. *BMJ Open* 2018 Apr;8(4):e018924. doi:10.1136/bmjopen-2017-018924
5. Saridogan E, Byrne D. The British Society for Gynaecological Endoscopy endometriosis centres project. *Gynecol Obstet Invest* 2013;76(1):10–13. doi:10.1159/000348520
6. Ugwumadu L, Chakrabarti R, Williams-Brown E, et al. The role of the multidisciplinary team in the management of deep infiltrating endometriosis. *Gynecol Surg* 2017;14(1):15. doi:10.1186/s10397-017-1018-0
7. Fang QY, Campbell N, Mooney SS, et al. Evidence for the role of multidisciplinary team care in people with pelvic pain and endometriosis: A systematic review. *Aust N Z J Obstet Gynaecol* 2023 Sep;ajo.13755. doi:10.1111/ajo.13755
8. Terho AM, Mäkelä-Kaikkonen J, Ohtonen P, et al. Robotic versus laparoscopic surgery for severe deep endometriosis: Protocol for a randomised controlled trial (ROBEndo trial). *BMJ Open* 2022 Jul;12(7):e063572. doi:10.1136/bmjopen-2022-063572
9. Magrina JF, Espada M, Kho RM, et al. Surgical excision of advanced endometriosis: Perioperative outcomes and impacting factors. *J Minim Invasive Gynecol* 2015 Sep;22(6):944–50. doi:10.1016/j.jmig.2015.04.016
10. Soto E, Luu TH, Liu X, et al. Laparoscopy vs. Robotic Surgery for Endometriosis (LAROSE): A multicenter, randomized, controlled trial. *Fertil Steril* 2017 Apr;107(4):996–1002.e3. doi:10.1016/j.fertnstert.2016.12.033
11. Nezhat CR, Stevens A, Balassiano E, et al. Robotic-assisted laparoscopy vs conventional laparoscopy for the treatment of advanced stage endometriosis. *J Minim Invasive Gynecol* 2015 Jan;22(1):40–4. doi:10.1016/j.jmig.2014.06.002
12. Le Gac M, Ferrier C, Touboul C, et al. Comparison of robotic versus conventional laparoscopy for the treatment of colorectal endometriosis: Pilot study of an expert center. *J Gynecol Obstet Hum Reprod* 2020 Dec;49(10):101885. doi:10.1016/j.jogoh.2020.101885

13. Ferrier C, Le Gas M, Kolanska K, et al. Comparison of robot-assisted and conventional laparoscopy for colorectal surgery for endometriosis: A prospective cohort study. *Int J Med Robot* 2022 Jun;18(3):e2382. doi:10.1002/rcs.2382

14. Gkegkes ID, Iavazzo C, Iatrakis G, et al. Robotic management of endometriosis: Discussion of use, criteria and advantages: A review of the literature. *Acta Medica Hradec Kralove Czech Repub* 2019;62(4):147–9. doi:10.14712/18059694.2020.3

15. Duffy JMN, Arambage K, Correa FJS, et al. Laparoscopic surgery for endometriosis. *Cochrane Database Syst Rev* 2014 Apr 3;3(4):CD011031; The Cochrane Collaboration, Ed., Chichester, UK: John Wiley & Sons, Ltd: p. CD011031.pub2. doi:10.1002/14651858.CD011031.pub2

16. Abbott J, Hawe J, Hunter D, et al. Laparoscopic excision of endometriosis: A randomized, placebo-controlled trial. *Fertil Steril* 2004 Oct;82(4):878–84. doi:10.1016/j.fertnstert.2004.03.046

17. Pundir J, Omanwa K, Kovoor E, et al. Laparoscopic excision versus ablation for endometriosis-associated pain: An updated systematic review and meta-analysis. *J Minim Invasive Gynecol* 2017;24(5):747–56. doi:10.1016/j.jmig.2017.04.008

18. Burks C, Lee M, DeSarno M, et al. Excision versus ablation for management of minimal to mild endometriosis: A systematic review and meta-analysis. *J Minim Invasive Gynecol* 2021 Mar;28(3):587–97. doi:10.1016/j.jmig.2020.11.028

19. Proctor ML, Latthe PM, Farquhar CM, et al. Surgical interruption of pelvic nerve pathways for primary and secondary dysmenorrhoea. *Cochrane Database Syst Rev* 2005 Oct;2005(4):CD001896. doi:10.1002/14651858.CD001896.pub2

20. Hart RJ, Hickey M, Maouris P, et al. Excisional surgery versus ablative surgery for ovarian endometriomata. *Cochrane Database Syst Rev* 2008 Apr;2:CD004992. doi:10.1002/14651858.CD004992.pub3

21. Candiani M, Ottolina J, Schimberni M, et al. Recurrence rate after 'one-step' CO2 fiber laser vaporization versus cystectomy for ovarian endometrioma: A 3-year follow-up study. *J Minim Invasive Gynecol* 2020 May;27(4):901–8. doi:10.1016/j.jmig.2019.07.027

22. Younis JS, Shapso N, Fleming R, et al. Impact of unilateral versus bilateral ovarian endometriotic cystectomy on ovarian reserve: A systematic review and meta-analysis. *Hum Reprod Update* 2019 May;25(3):375–91. doi:10.1093/humupd/dmy049

23. Muzii L, Achilli C, Lecce F, et al. Second surgery for recurrent endometriomas is more harmful to healthy ovarian tissue and ovarian reserve than first surgery. *Fertil Steril* 2015 Mar;103(3):738–43. doi:10.1016/j.fertnstert.2014.12.101

24. Busacca M, Riparini J, Somigliana E, et al. Postsurgical ovarian failure after laparoscopic excision of bilateral endometriomas. *Am J Obstet Gynecol* 2006 Aug;195(2):421–5. doi:10.1016/j.ajog.2006.03.064

25. Wills HJ, Reid GD, Cooper MJW, et al. Fertility and pain outcomes following laparoscopic segmental bowel resection for colorectal endometriosis: A review. *Aust N Z J Obstet Gynaecol* 208 Jun;48(3):292–5. doi:10.1111/j.1479-828X.2008.00871.x

26. Vercellini P, Somigliana E, Consonni D, et al. Surgical versus medical treatment for endometriosis-associated severe deep dyspareunia: I. Effect on pain during intercourse and patient satisfaction. *Hum Reprod Oxf Engl* 2012 Ded;27(12):3450–9. doi:10.1093/humrep/des313

27. Sandström A, Bixo M, Johansson M, et al. Effect of hysterectomy on pain in women with endometriosis: A population-based registry study. *BJOG Int J Obstet Gynaecol* 2020 Dec;127(13):1628–35. doi:10.1111/1471-0528.16328

28. Martin DC. Hysterectomy for treatment of pain associated with endometriosis. *J Minim Invasive Gynecol* 2006;13(6):566–72. doi:10.1016/j.jmig.2006.06.022

29. Shakiba K, Bena JF, McGill KM, et al. Surgical treatment of endometriosis: A 7-year follow-up on the requirement for further surgery. *Obstet Gynecol* 2008 Jun;111(6):1285–92. doi:10.1097/AOG.0b013e3181758ec6; Contraceptive for pelvic pain associated with endometriosis. *Fertil Steril* 1993 Jul;60(1):75–79.

30. Sandström A, Bixo M, Johansson M, et al. Effect of hysterectomy on pain in women with endometriosis: A population-based registry study. *BJOG* 2020;127:1628–35. doi:10.1111/1471-0528.16328 pmid:32437082 [CrossRef] [PubMed] [Google Scholar]

31. Shakiba K, Bena JF, McGill KM, et al. Surgical treatment of endometriosis: A 7-year follow-up on the requirement for further surgery. *Obstet Gynecol* 2008;111:1285–92. doi:10.1097/AOG.0b013e3181758ec6 pmid:18515510 [CrossRef] [PubMed] [Web of Science] [Google Scholar]

32. Orlando MS, Luna Russo MA, Richards EG, et al. Racial and ethnic disparities in surgical care for endometriosis across the United States. *Am J Obstet Gynecol* 2022;226:824.e1–11. doi:10.1016/j.ajog.2022.01.021 pmid:35101410

33. Stewart EA, Missmer SA, Rocca WA. Moving beyond reflexive and prophylactic gynecologic surgery. *Mayo Clin Proc* 2021;96:291–4. doi:10.1016/j.mayocp.2020.05.012 pmid:33549251 [CrossRef] [PubMed] [Google Scholar]

34. Mu F, Rich-Edwards J, Rimm EB, et al. Endometriosis and risk of coronary heart disease. *Circ Cardiovasc Qual Outcomes* 2016;9:257–64. doi:10.1161/CIRCOUTCOMES.115.002224 pmid:27025928 [Abstract/FREE Full Text] [Google Scholar]

35. Laughlin-Tommaso SK, Khan Z, Weaver AL, et al. Cardiovascular and metabolic morbidity after hysterectomy with ovarian conservation: A cohort study. *Menopause* 2018;25:483–92. doi:10.1097/GME.0000000000001043 pmid:29286988 [CrossRef] [PubMed] [Google Scholar]

36. Hans Evers JL. Is adolescent endometriosis a progressive disease that needs to be diagnosed and treated? *Hum Reprod* 2013;28:2023. doi:10.1093/humrep/det298 pmid:23861497 [CrossRef] [PubMed] [Google Scholar]

37. As-Sanie S, Till SR, Schrepf AD, et al. Incidence and predictors of persistent pelvic pain following hysterectomy in women with chronic pelvic pain. *Am J Obstet Gynecol* 2021;225:568.e1–11. doi:10.1016/j.ajog.2021.08.038 pmid:34464585 [CrossRef] [PubMed] [Google Scholar]

38. Chen I, Veth VB, Choudhry AJ, et al. Pre- and postsurgical medical therapy for endometriosis surgery. *Cochrane Database Syst Rev* 2020;11:CD003678. pmid:33206374 [PubMed] [Google Scholar]

39. British Menopause Society. *Tools for clinicians: Induced menopause in women with endometriosis.* 2019. https://thebms.org.uk/publications/tools-for-clinicians/

FURTHER READING

BSGE. *Endometriosis centres subcommittee.* [Online]. www.bsge.org.uk/committees/endometriosis-centres/ (accessed 11 Oct 2023).

ESHRE. *Endometriosis by the European Society of Human Reproduction and Embryology.* ESHRE. [Online]. www.eshre.eu/Guideline/Endometriosis (accessed 22 Nov 2023).

NICE. *Endometriosis: Diagnosis and management.* [Online]. www.nice.org.uk/guidance/ng73 (accessed 22 Nov 2023).

CHAPTER 10B

Surgical Management II

....

Hannah Draper and Andrew Horne

INTRODUCTION

Surgery remains an important way to both definitively diagnose and treat endometriosis. Women may opt for laparoscopy to gain a definitive diagnosis, treat pain symptoms or as part of fertility treatment. Until more effective medical options for the treatment for endometriosis are developed, surgery will remain as a cornerstone of treatment. This chapter aims to provide an overview of the surgical management of endometriosis currently provided in the UK.

REFERRAL TO SECONDARY CARE

Women with endometriosis still wait on average 8 years for a diagnosis and will often have ongoing symptoms long after this. Current NICE guidance states that women should be referred to gynaecology services if they have severe, persistent or recurrent symptoms of endometriosis; pelvic signs of endometriosis; or initial management is not effective, not tolerated or contraindicated (1,2). In practice, many women with endometriosis symptoms will often wish referral at this stage. By the time that women are referred to secondary care, they will usually have trialled at least one hormonal treatment and be keen to explore what surgical options are available.

Some women will have endometriosis involving their bowel, bladder or ureter diagnosed on imaging performed in primary care. If this is suspected, or there is a suspicion of endometriosis outside the pelvic

DOI: 10.1201/9781032684819-12

cavity, they should be referred directly to one of the network of specialist endometriosis centres where there is expertise in the diagnosis and management of endometriosis including advanced laparoscopic surgical skills (see www.bsge.org.uk). A specialist centre comprises a multidisciplinary team that includes both colorectal and urological surgeons with an interest in endometriosis, an endometriosis specialist nurse, pain management service with expertise in pelvic pain, experts in gynaecological imaging of endometriosis, advanced diagnostic facilities and fertility services. Endometriosis is a chronic, systemic disease where untreated disease can result in significant end organ damage such as bowel or ureteric obstruction. It is, therefore, vital that women with severe disease have access to expert multidisciplinary care as soon as possible.

Endometriosis has a high prevalence among adolescent girls with pelvic pain. Since this is a condition which may well affect them for the rest of their life, any patient under 17 who you suspect to have endometriosis should be referred to secondary care (1). Whether this is a general gynaecology service, paediatric and adolescent gynaecology service or endometriosis centre will depend on local service provisions.

Some women will have confirmed endometriosis but choose not to undergo surgery. They should receive their follow-up in secondary care especially if they have an endometrioma larger than 3 cm or they have deep endometriosis involving the bowel, bladder or ureter (1).

CHOOSING TO UNDERGO SURGERY

The decision to undergo surgery should be through a shared approach between the surgeon and patient. This is likely to be a very individual decision which includes considerations such as treatment aims and the patient's wishes for future fertility. The surgical management of endometriosis encompasses a spectrum of surgery from straightforward laparoscopic excision and/or ablation to complex surgery which may involve urological or colorectal surgeons. The reasons that women choose to undergo surgery will be similarly varied from gaining a definitive diagnosis, to pain management or as part of fertility treatment. For this reason, when patients are referred to secondary care, they should have an initial consultation with a gynaecologist who can explore their symptoms, preferences and priorities, which may include pain management and future fertility. These are the cornerstones which guide decision-making around surgery and should be a shared approach between the surgeon and patient.

The current guidelines by both NICE (1) and ESHRE (3) recommend surgery as a treatment option for the management of endometriosis-associated pain. However, the studies on which these recommendations are based tend to amalgamate all subtypes of endometriosis and have relatively short follow-up periods (4). The evidence supporting an improvement in pain or quality of life is often based on low-quality studies. The benefits of surgery are likely to be dependent on the subtype of endometriosis and the desired outcomes such as pain management or treatment of fertility. Unfortunately, there are currently no prognostic markers that can be used to select who will benefit most from surgery (3).

SURGERY FOR DIAGNOSIS

Many patients attending primary care will have symptoms which suggest endometriosis but have no obvious pathology found on imaging and whose symptoms do not resolve with empirical therapy. In these patients, a diagnostic laparoscopy is recommended by both NICE (1) and ESHRE (3). This is usually performed as a day case and should involve a systematic visual assessment of the abdominal and pelvic cavity. Histological confirmation of endometriosis remains the gold standard; however, it does not have a particularly high sensitivity particularly in young women (5,6).

Endometriosis can have a variety of surgical appearances from black or dark blue "spots," through white opacifications to red flame-like lesions and yellow "patches" (Figure 10B.1). Ovarian endometriomas

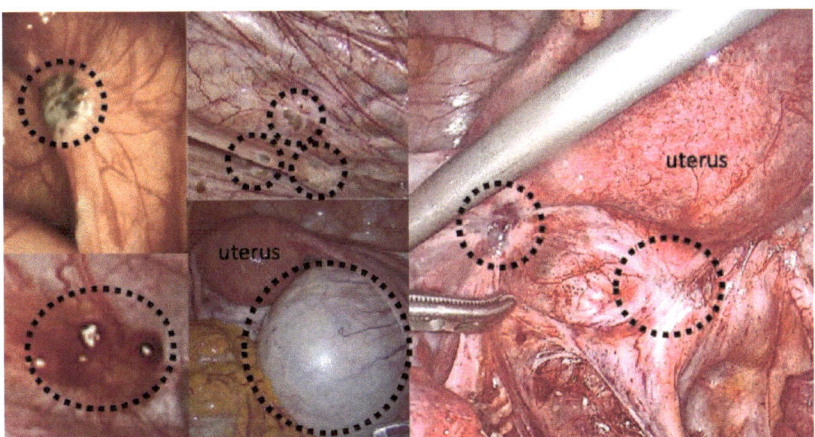

FIGURE 10B.1 Surgical images of the types of endometriosis. (Image reproduced courtesy of Andrew Horne and Stacey Missmer [2].)

have a distinct appearance and are often described as "chocolate cysts" due to their dark brown appearance as a result of collections of menstrual blood and necrotic fluid. Deep endometriosis is often found as multifocal nodules which invade any of the surrounding peritoneum and viscera. Endometriosis is also associated with both adhesions and fibrotic scar tissue and is often found where ovaries are fixed by adhesions (7). There remains a high rate of laparoscopies where no underlying pathology is found and is thought to be as high as 40% (8). As with any investigation, it relies on the skill and experience of the individual, but women should be reassured that a negative laparoscopy performed by an experienced surgeon is highly sensitive (9).

THERAPEUTIC SURGERY

When endometriosis is found during a diagnostic laparoscopy, it can be managed on a "see and treat basis," or, where this is not possible, it should be adequately described to allow future surgical planning or refer-ral to an endometriosis specialist centre for ongoing care. The aims of surgery are primarily to remove or treat all visible endometriosis and to restore the pelvic anatomy which may have been distorted by adhesions.

There are primarily two approaches to the treatment of endometrio-sis deposits: They can either be ablated using heat or laser, which aims to destroy endometriosis lesions, or they can be excised. Surgeons may often use a combination of these techniques dependent on the type and location of the lesions. Most patients will wish, especially initially, for conservative treatment, which may involve resection of lesions but with preservation of the ovaries and uterus.

Perhaps the greatest debate for the benefit of surgery surrounds the surgical treatment of superficial peritoneal endometriosis. There is lit-tle evidence to suggest that it improves either symptoms or quality of life. In addition, the available evidence does not allow us to understand whether ablation and excision have comparable results and, therefore, make an informed decision about the type of operation that should be performed (10,11). Many patients with superficial peritoneal endome-triosis will undergo multiple therapeutic laparoscopies and the risks and possible long-term harm associated with postoperative scarring need to be considered.

Patients with endometrioma are usually offered surgical management, although there is not a large evidence base to support this over a conserv-ative approach. The risk of recurrence of both the endometrioma and its associated pain is reduced if cysts are excised rather than drained and ablated (12). This also allows for a histological diagnosis of the cyst wall to exclude malignancy. For those who wish for future fertility, a cautious approach should be used to aim to conserve ovarian reserve and to avoid damage to healthy ovarian tissue (13). Many clinicians will often avoid performing a cystectomy and opt for drainage in these patients.

SURGERY FOR DEEP ENDOMETRIOSIS

Deep endometriosis can involve extensive adhesions and fibrosis surrounding endometriosis deposits creating large nodules involving adjacent structures such as the bowel, bladder or ureter. Currently, the best treatment is generally considered to be laparoscopic surgery to completely excise all disease. There are a number of studies which demonstrate both statistically and clinically significant improvement of symptoms including pain, dyspareunia, dyschezia and quality of life (2). Studies evaluating this approach are often limited by being performed in single centres or not including control arms for comparison. However, a large multicentre study undertaken in BSGE-accredited endometriosis centres demonstrated that women who had rectovaginal nodules excised had significant improvement in their pelvic pain and bowel symptoms. There was a significant improvement in reported health-related quality of life measures which lasted for the 2-year follow-up period (14).

Surgery for deep endometriosis can include a broad range of different surgical procedures. Deep endometriosis most commonly invades the ovaries, fallopian tubes, pelvic sidewalls, bladder and bowel. In addition to the endometriosis lesions, there can be significant adhesions adhering the pelvic organs which can significantly distort the anatomy. These adhesions can cause bowel or ureteric obstruction which will not respond to medical therapy due to irreversible fibrosis (15). In order to safely treat both the endometriosis and adhesions, these procedures are commonly performed jointly with urologists and colorectal surgeons and should be performed in specialist endometriosis centres. Women with deep endometriosis will often have scar tissue and endometriosis that attaches the bowel, bladder and other structures together. The surgical planes and anatomy can be completely distorted, requiring meticulous and careful dissection to prevent damaging other structures.

Bowel endometriosis is thought to affect 5–30% of women with endometriosis and can be treated in a variety of ways dependent on how deeply the endometriosis has invaded and the anatomical location of the nodules (16). It is usually performed jointly with colorectal surgeons or gynaecologists with additional training. Patients need to be carefully counselled about both the recovery and potential risks of these, particularly when future fertility is desired (3). Although preoperative planning with MRI or ultrasound can be helpful, it is often uncertain how deeply a nodule invades into the surface of the bowel until the disease is actually being removed. Sometimes all visible endometriosis can be removed by carefully shaving it off the surface of the bowel without damage (shave), occasionally a small area of bowel is removed and closed (disc resection), but for complex disease, a segmental resection with or without a temporary stoma is required. Where bowel endometriosis is suspected, women are usually counselled about all options including temporary stoma, and if it is found unexpectedly, a second stage procedure would be arranged. Women can often feel very isolated during recovery from bowel surgery and can often have symptoms of anterior resection syndrome especially initially. These can include faecal frequency, urgency and occasional episodes of leakage or incontinence.

Cystoscopy and the placement of temporary ureteric stents can be performed to both help the relevant surgeons to safely identify the ureters intra-operatively to reduce the risk of damage and prevent postoperative obstruction if ureterolysis is performed. Rarely, more complex urological procedures such as nephrectomy or reimplantation of ureters are necessary, but this would only be offered following multidisciplinary discussions and counselling of the patient.

HYSTERECTOMY

Whilst hysterectomy is not a recognized cure for endometriosis, it remains a treatment option for some women, particularly those who have co-existing adenomyosis and those who have exhausted all other alternative treatments (17). NICE recommends that hysterectomy can be offered to women who do not wish to conceive and who have trialled more conservative treatment without success. The majority of hysterectomies performed for endometriosis will be laparoscopic (or laparoscopically-assisted) total hysterectomies (17). The cervix is usually removed to both prevent any breakthrough bleeding and reduce the possibility of residual endometrium. However, this may not always be possible and either a subtotal hysterectomy (preservation of the cervix) or an open procedure is required. Whether the ovaries are removed or not, the aim should be to remove all visible endometriosis at the time of hysterectomy (1,3).

Both NICE and ESHRE recommend that when considering removing the ovaries, the long-term consequence of early menopause and possible need for HRT should be considered. Currently available longitudinal studies show that for long-term management of pain, removal of the ovaries does not have an additional benefit over ovarian conservation (17,18). In addition to the sudden onset of menopausal symptoms, the long-term risks of early surgical menopause are well-documented and include osteoporosis, cardiovascular disease and sexual dysfunction. These can be improved with the use of HRT, but long-term systemic effects of surgical menopause are not yet fully understood. The decision as to whether to remove the ovaries will be dependent on the woman's wishes as well as her age and other risk factors such as family history of malignancy.

Ovarian preservation does not necessarily protect women from long-term morbidity including cardiovascular and metabolic disease (19) as well as new onset depression (20). These risks are particularly prominent in women aged under 35 at the time of surgery. The surgical risks of laparoscopic hysterectomy for endometriosis include infection; bleeding requiring a blood transfusion; damage to internal organs such as bowel, bladder, ureters and blood vessels; venous thromboembolism; hernia formation; and the need to convert to an open procedure. The surgical risks for those with mild–moderate endometriosis are similar to the general population (21), but for those with severe endometriosis, there is a greater chance of longer operating time and major complication (21,22). It should also be noted that despite the fact that endometriosis has an estimated 10% prevalence among all reproductive-aged women, the incidence of complications remains higher in BIPOC women (23). All patients undergoing surgery for endometriosis should be counselled that there is a chance that symptoms will either fail to resolve or will recur in the future.

Whilst for many women these risks will be acceptable when balanced against intractable pain and other endometriosis symptoms, they need to be fully discussed and carefully considered on an individual basis.

SURGERY FOR RECURRENT SYMPTOMS

The management of recurrent endometriosis symptoms can be challenging. It is estimated that after surgical treatment, 21.5% of women will report recurrence of painful symptoms at 2 years and up to 50% at 5 years (18,24). This is compounded by our lack of understanding about the natural history of the disease where it is likely that some lesions will regress, some remain static, and the remainder will progress (25). We do not have any ability to currently predict which lesions are which and offer tailored treatment. There is also a concern that repeated surgical treatment may worsen symptoms for some women, and medical management of symptoms should also be considered. It should be noted that the recurrence of symptoms does not always mean that the disease has recurred, and the impact of adenomyosis and central pain sensitization should be considered. Women who have recurrent or intractable symptoms should be referred to specialist endometriosis centres for expert management (1).

ENDOMETRIOSIS CENTRES AND MULTIDISCIPLINARY APPROACH

Specialist endometriosis centres were first introduced in the UK in 2006 (see BSGE website). Whilst they allow patients to access expert surgeons with additional training in advanced laparoscopic skills, they are also designed to provide holistic coordinated care. There is an increasing understanding that the symptoms of endometriosis can not only be complex but can evolve across a woman's life. It is, therefore, vital that women receive multidisciplinary care from clinicians including colorectal and urological surgeons, pain medicine specialists, endometriosis specialist nurses, experts in imaging, fertility specialists, psychologists and physiotherapists. Patients can usually be directly referred from primary care as well as by gynaecologists, and this should be considered early, particularly in patients who are believed to have deep or extra-abdominal endometriosis (3).

SECONDARY PREVENTION

For patients who do not wish for immediate fertility, many clinicians will offer postoperative hormonal therapy as secondary prevention. There is evidence to support the use of a levonorgestrel-releasing intrauterine system or combined hormonal contraceptive for 18–24 months postoperatively to reduce dysmenorrhea (26). These are also recommended by ESHRE to prevent the recurrence of ovarian endometrioma and its associated symptoms (3).

Patients who undergo surgical menopause should receive combined HRT rather than oestrogen-only preparations until at least the age of natural menopause (3). The addition of progesterone aims to reduce both the risk of recurrence and malignant transformation. Endometriosis can remain active and cause symptoms after the menopause. Where women require HRT after either natural or surgical menopause, combined oestrogen and progesterone preparations should be used (3). For those who undergo the surgical menopause, this should continue until at least the age of the natural menopause (3). There is a higher risk of malignant transformation in women with a history of endometriosis who receive oestrogen-only treatments for vasomotor symptoms, so this should be avoided (27).

SURGICAL MANAGEMENT IF FERTILITY IS A PRIORITY

Approximately 30–50% of women with endometriosis will experience fertility problems; however, the underlying mechanisms which cause endometriosis-related infertility remain elusive (28). Many patients with endometriosis will have disordered pelvic anatomy with significant adhesions that can cause a mechanical obstacle preventing fertilization. The options for patients are primarily expectant, surgery or assisted reproductive techniques. When patients are older or where it is suspected that they have extensive disease, it may be better to reduce the length of expectant management.

The aim of surgery in this situation is to normalize the pelvic anatomy (or improve it as far as possible) as well as to remove endometriotic tissue. Endometriosis has an effect on fertility and pregnancy which cannot simply be explained by mechanical obstruction alone, and there is an increased incidence of both miscarriage and adverse obstetric outcomes. There are likely to be molecular processes which could affect both oocyte quality and endometrial receptivity. It is possible that ovaries may be damaged due to surgery or directly by toxic effects of endometriosis (29). The factors underpinning infertility caused by endometriosis are not yet truly understood, and this should be considered when counselling patients about the benefits of surgery. There is only a modest improvement in spontaneous pregnancy rates after removal of endometriosis lesions but it is recommended by NICE in women where their endometriosis does not affect their bowel, bladder or ureter because of an increase in spontaneous conception (1). They also recommend excision of endometriomas to reduce the risk of recurrence and improve the chance of pregnancy; however, they note that caution should be taken of damaging ovarian reserve (1).

The role of surgery prior to assisted reproductive technology (ART) remains controversial. Whilst some patients will require surgery to improve their pain or to ensure that their follicles are safely accessible, it is not currently routinely recommended by ESHRE due to a lack of evidence about its efficacy. The risks of surgery should be balanced against the possible benefits, which may be modest. It is possible that surgery may not restore pelvic anatomy, new adhesions may form and ovarian reserve may be reduced. For women with deep endometriosis affecting their bowel, bladder or ureter, surgical treatment needs to be planned in conjunction with both fertility and endometriosis teams. The benefits of surgery in these patients may be less than those with less severe disease and the risk of a major complications such as a bowel resection need to be weighed against any potential benefit. Currently, surgery should be reserved for those with painful symptoms.

The Endometriosis Fertility Index (EFI) has been developed to help to predict spontaneous pregnancy rates in patients with surgically proven endometriosis and includes factors such as age, duration of infertility, pregnancy history, endometriosis severity and surgical appearances (30). It can be a useful tool to provide tailored counselling and management to couples experiencing infertility.

KEY POINT SUMMARY

- Surgery remains one of the key management options for women with endometriosis, but it is not a definitive treatment for many women.
- Early referral of women with deep endometriosis to specialist endometriosis centres will allow them to access the expert multidisciplinary care that they will require to manage their complex symptoms.
- Endometriosis may account for up to 40% of pelvic pain in adolescent girls, and anyone under the age of 17 who is suspected to have endometriosis should be referred directly to secondary care.
- Endometriosis should be considered as a cause of recurrent symptoms even after a hysterectomy or menopause, and referral to secondary care should be considered.
- HRT can be offered to women with endometriosis who are going through the surgical or natural menopause. Continuous combined HRT should be offered to reduce the risk of endometriosis recurrence and malignant transformation.

REFERENCES

1. Diagnosis and management of endometriosis: Summary of NICE guidance. *BMJ* 2017;j4227.
2. Horne AW, Missmer SA. Pathophysiology, diagnosis, and management of endometriosis. *BMJ* 2022;379:e070750.
3. Becker CM, Bokor A, Heikinheimo O, et al. ESHRE guideline: Endometriosis. *Hum Reprod Open* 2022;2022(2):hoac009.

4. Bafort C, Beebeejaun Y, Tomassetti C, et al. Laparoscopic surgery for endometriosis. *Cochrane Database of Syst Rev* 2020;10.

5. Watkins JC, DiVasta AD, Vitonis AF, et al. A clinical and pathologic exploration of suspected peritoneal endometriotic lesions. *Int J Gynecol Pathol* 2021;40(6):602–10.

6. Taylor HS, Adamson GD, Diamond MP, et al. An evidence-based approach to assessing surgical versus clinical diagnosis of symptomatic endometriosis. *Int J Gynaecol Obstet* 2018;142(2):131–42.

7. Rao T, Condous G, Reid S. Ovarian immobility at transvaginal ultrasound: An important sonographic marker for prediction of need for pelvic side-wall surgery in women with suspected endometriosis. *J Ultrasound Med* 2022;41(5):1109–13.

8. Lamvu G, Carrillo J, Ouyang C, et al. Chronic pelvic pain in women: A review. *JAMA* 2021;325(23):2381–91.

9. Wykes CB, Clark TJ, Khan KS. Accuracy of laparoscopy in the diagnosis of endometriosis: A systematic quantitative review. *BJOG* 2004;111(11):1204–12.

10. Burks C, Lee M, DeSarno M, et al. Excision versus ablation for management of minimal to mild endometriosis: A systematic review and meta-analysis. *J Minim Invasive Gynecol* 2021;28(3):587–97.

11. Pundir J, Omanwa K, Kovoor E, et al. Laparoscopic excision versus ablation for endometriosis-associated pain: An updated systematic review and meta-analysis. *J Minim Invasive Gynecol* 2017;24(5):747–56.

12. Hart RJ, Hickey M, Maouris P, et al. Excisional surgery versus ablative surgery for ovarian endometriomata. *Cochrane Database Syst Rev* 2008(2):Cd004992.

13. Shaltout MF, Elsheikhah A, Maged AM, et al. A randomized controlled trial of a new technique for laparoscopic management of ovarian endometriosis preventing recurrence and keeping ovarian reserve. *J Ovarian Res* 2019;12(1):66.

14. Byrne D, Curnow T, Smith P, et al. Laparoscopic excision of deep rectovaginal endometriosis in BSGE endometriosis centres: A multicentre prospective cohort study. *BMJ Open* 2018;8(4):e018924.

15. Zanelotti A, Decherney AH. Surgery and endometriosis. *Clin Obstet Gynecol* 2017;60(3):477–84.

16. Nezhat C, Li Anjie, Falik R, Nezhat A, Nazhat C, et al. Bowel endometriosis: Diagnosis and management. *Am J Obstet Gynecol* 218(6):549–62. doi:10.1016/j.ajog.2017.09.023

17. Sandström A, Bixo M, Johansson M, et al. Effect of hysterectomy on pain in women with endometriosis: A population-based registry study. *BJOG: Int J Obstet Gynaecol* 2020;127(13):1628–35.

18. Shakiba K, Bena JF, McGill KM, et al. Surgical treatment of endometriosis: A 7-year follow-up on the requirement for further surgery. *Obstet Gynecol* 2008;111(6):1285–92.

19. Laughlin-Tommaso SK, Khan Z, Weaver AL, et al. Cardiovascular and metabolic morbidity after hysterectomy with ovarian conservation: A cohort study. *Menopause* 2018;25(5):483–92.

20. Laughlin-Tommaso SK, Satish A, Khan Z, et al. Long-term risk of de novo mental health conditions after hysterectomy with ovarian conservation: A cohort study. *Menopause* 2020;27(1):33–42.

21. Uccella S, Marconi N, Casarin J, et al. Impact of endometriosis on surgical outcomes and complications of total laparoscopic hysterectomy. *Arch Gynecol Obstet* 2016;294(4):771–8.

22. Stewart KA, Tessier KM, Lebovic DI. Comparing characteristics of and postoperative morbidity after hysterectomy for endometriosis versus other benign indications: A NSQIP study. *J Minim Invasive Gynecol* 2022;29(7):884–90.e2.
23. Orlando MS, Luna Russo MA, Richards EG, et al. Racial and ethnic disparities in surgical care for endometriosis across the United States. *Am J Obstet Gynecol* 2022;226(6):824.e1–11.
24. Guo SW. Recurrence of endometriosis and its control. *Hum Reprod Update* 2009;15(4):441–61.
25. Evers JLH. Is adolescent endometriosis a progressive disease that needs to be diagnosed and treated? *Hum Reprod* 2013;28(8):2023.
26. Chen I, Veth VB, Choudhry AJ, et al. Pre- and postsurgical medical therapy for endometriosis surgery. *Cochrane Database Syst Rev* 2020;11(11):Cd003678.
27. Gemmell LC, Webster KE, Kirtley S, et al. The management of menopause in women with a history of endometriosis: A systematic review. *Hum Reprod Update* 2017;23(4):481–500.
28. Zondervan KT, Becker CM, Koga K, et al. Endometriosis. *Nat Rev Dis Primers* 2018;4(1):9.
29. Senapati S, Sammel MD, Morse C, et al. Impact of endometriosis on in vitro fertilization outcomes: An evaluation of the society for assisted reproductive technologies database. *Fertil Steril* 2016;106(1):164–71.e1.
30. Adamson GD, Pasta DJ. Endometriosis fertility index: The new, validated endometriosis staging system. *Fertil Steril* 2010;94(5):1609–15.

FURTHER READING

BSGE. *Endometriosis centres subcommittee.* [Online]. www.bsge.org.uk/committees/endometriosis-centres/ (accessed 11 Oct 2023).
ESHRE. *Endometriosis by the European Society of Human Reproduction and Embryology.* ESHRE. [Online]. www.eshre.eu/Guideline/Endometriosis (accessed 22 Nov 2023).
NICE. *Endometriosis: Diagnosis and management.* [Online]. www.nice.org.uk/guidance/ng73 (accessed 22 Nov 2023).

CHAPTER 11

Tertiary Care: The Specialist Endometriosis Centre

....

Levels of care refer to the complexity of medical cases, the types of conditions a physician treats and their specialties.

The levels of care are: Primary, secondary, tertiary and quaternary care. Sometimes problems arise in secondary care due to:

- *Referral to a wrong specialist*: That can happen because symptoms often overlap between a variety of health conditions, for example, endometriosis, heavy menstrual bleed and infertility. The symptoms suggest one problem, but the referral is sent to a different specialist

- *Lack of coordination of care*: This happens when a patient is seen by more than one specialist, and each is focusing on a different issue. The treatment of endometriosis depends on the type and severity of symptoms, whether the patient is planning for a pregnancy and personal preferences to treatment. In situations where initial pain-relieving medications have not been helpful, referral is done to a specialist pain management team that may include physiotherapists and psychologists. Hormonal treatments to control bleeding and pain include combined oral contraceptive pill or GnRH given as injection. Not all secondary care hospitals provide gonadotropin-releasing hormone (GnRH) agonists

SPECIALIST ENDOMETRIOSIS CENTRE

This is a higher level of specialized care. It requires highly specialized equipment and expertise. A local hospital is not able to provide this care.

DOI: 10.1201/9781032684819-13

A Specialist Endometriosis Centre is also called tertiary care.

Quaternary care: This is considered an extension of tertiary care. It is more specialized and highly unusual, for example, uncommon and specialized surgery and some types of uncommon diagnostic and experimental medicine.

Specialist centres were first formally proposed in 2006 (1), and this model of care has been successfully implemented in the UK and several other European countries such as Denmark, Germany and France (2,3).

The role of specialist endometriosis centres should be to offer a coordinated, holistic, multidisciplinary, multimodal approach to women with complex symptoms of endometriosis. Although relevant surgical expertise is important, the role of a centre is not to focus solely on surgical treatment to eradicate lesions but to offer an integrated service, including gynaecologists, colorectal surgeons, urologists, endometriosis specialist nurses, pain medicine specialists, psychologists, physiotherapists, fertility specialists and imaging experts.

Endometriosis Diagnosis and Management: NICE Guideline (NG73) recognizes the British Society for Gynaecological Endoscopy (BSGE) endometriosis centres. They are seen as an opportunity to deliver a specialist service nationally which should prove to be beneficial to patients and more cost effective.

Specialist Endometriosis Centre

Specialist Endometriosis Centres should have access to:

- Gynaecologists with expertise in diagnosing and managing endometriosis, including advanced laparoscopic surgical skills
- Colorectal surgeon with an interest in endometriosis
- Urologist with an interest in endometriosis
- Thoracic surgeon
- Endometriosis specialist nurse
- Multidisciplinary pain management service with expertise in pelvic pain
- Health care professional with specialist expertise in gynaecological imaging of endometriosis
- Advanced diagnostic facilities (for example, radiology and histopathology)
- Fertility services

AIMS OF THE SPECIALIST ENDOMETRIOSIS CENTRE

The aim of the specialist endometriosis centre is to provide patient-centred specialist care for women with severe endometriosis, improving their quality of life as per NHS Outcomes Framework Domains and Indicators by:

- Clearly defining and explaining the extent of the disease
- Providing appropriate counselling and psychological support
- Providing a nurse specialist who will interface between patient and specialist team
- Individualizing care based on the patient's specific symptom complex and preferences
- Taking account of the patient's fertility needs
- Providing high-quality treatment and care to relieve symptoms of endometriosis
- Assessing quality of life before and, at intervals, after treatment

---

NHS Outcomes Framework Domains and Indicators

Domain 1 Preventing people from dying prematurely.

Domain 2 Enhancing quality of life for people with long-term conditions.

Domain 3 Helping people to recover from episodes of ill-health or following injury.

Domain 4 Ensuring people have a positive experience of care.

Domain 5 Treating and caring for people in safe environment and protecting them from avoidable harm.

Referral to the Specialist Endometriosis Centre

- If the patient is suspected to have severe endometriosis based on certain symptoms, clinical examination or imaging or due to detection during previous surgery, patient should be referred to an endometriosis specialist centre. When endometriosis is severe, it affects more areas within the pelvis and abdomen, such as ovaries, bladder and bowel. Adhesions develop when scar tissue attaches separate structures or organs together causing severe and debilitating symptoms

- During clinical examination, if there is tenderness, nodules felt in the vaginal wall or seen during speculum examination, may favour deep endometriosis or endometriosis of ovaries. A transvaginal scan (TVS) may aid in the diagnosis of ovarian endometrioma or deep endometriosis. Women suspected to have severe endometriosis can have lesions on other organs or adhesions

- Patient requires fertility treatment. The tertiary centre closely collaborates with its in vitro fertilization (IVF) clinic, offering advanced fertility treatments including oocyte donation and gestational surrogacy

- Patient requiring integrated pain management

The specialist centre may request an MRI scan to assess the extent of the disease and/or additional imaging for assessment of the ureters, bladder and bowel involvement. It is a good idea to make sure that the following are done to avoid a rejected referral:

- Transvaginal scan
- MRI scan if suspicion of deep endometriosis on examination and USS showed large endometrioma of features of hydronephrosis
- Laparoscopy if pelvic USS and MRI were normal

Criteria for Surgical Management of Endometriosis in the Specialist Endometriosis Centre

- Complex or deep endometriosis involving bowel, bladder or ureters (confirmed at laparoscopy) in those wishing surgical treatment
- Extra pelvic endometriosis (such as but not limited to diaphragmatic or thoracic endometriosis) confirmed at laparoscopy or imaging (MRI/CT)
- BMI less than 35

> For any complex endometriosis cases that do not meet the prior criteria, patient should be discussed in the regional centre on an individual case basis.

MANAGEMENT OF PATIENTS IN THE SPECIALIST ENDOMETRIOSIS CENTRE

Every case is discussed in an endometriosis multidisciplinary team (MDT) meeting where all the specialists review the case and plan the management. The goal is to remove all endometriosis and relieve symptoms of the disease whilst incurring the lowest possible morbidity. The service will achieve this aim by:

- Providing complex laparoscopic surgical excision of all endometrioses irrespective of site
- Operating jointly, as required, with a second gynaecologist, a named colorectal surgeon and/or urologist

- Retaining pelvic structures unless there is an objective reason to remove them
- Maintaining a detailed surgical database to include detail of surgery and any complications
- Recording patient reported outcome measures (PROMs) on relevant clinical domains and quality of life
- Working with pain management specialists
- Keeping the use of open surgery to the minimum

What Are the Advantages of Centralized Care for Severe Endometriosis?

For many years, BSGE has championed the treatment for people with severe complex endometriosis to be performed in a centre where a large volume of similar cases are seen and a multidisciplinary team of specialists are accessible to the patient.

In a tertiary centre, the diagnosis and treatment are managed by a multidisciplinary team and care is managed faster.

What Does Surgery for Severe Endometriosis Involve?

With the aim of safely removing as much visible endometriosis as one can, the surgery usually involves:

- Removing any ovarian endometriotic cysts (endometriomas) and/or releasing the ovaries that may be stuck to the pelvic wall, uterus or to each other
- Dividing adhesions or scar tissues
- Identifying the ureters and freeing them by dissecting any endometriotic tissues around them
- Removing any tissue affected by endometriosis around the back and the side of the uterus, the ureter and the bladder, the space between the vagina and rectum or the bowel wall itself

Bowel Endometriosis

A specialist gynaecologist will perform the surgery if endometriosis has affected the bowel, which may be assisted by a bowel surgeon. The endometriotic tissue that has grown in the bowel is removed by:

- Shaving the lesions if the superficial surface of the bowel in involved
- Segmental resection, where a segment/section of the bowel is removed and the ends are joined together with metal staples

- Discoid resection, where a small "disc" of the bowel wall is removed and the defect is sutured

The type of surgery performed depends on area of bowel involved and extent of involvement. There is a potential risk of needing a temporary stoma to allow the bowel to heal. A stoma is a diversion of the bowel into a separate bag through an opening in the skin.

If a portion of the bowel is removed, patient will notice changes in the bowel movements such as going to the toilet more often and occasional incontinence. It usually takes few months for the bowel function to improve.

Bladder Endometriosis

A urologist (bladder surgeon) may help the specialist gynaecologist during the surgery if endometriosis affects the bladder and/or ureters.

If endometriosis involves the bladder, one may need a partial or full cystoscopy to see the extent of involvement. If a ureter is affected, one may need stenting (insertion of a small plastic tubes) and excision of ureteral lesions.

Risks of Surgery for Severe Endometriosis

Surgery for severe endometriosis is more complex and can be associated with complications with a high risk of injury to organs such as:

- Bowel injury, bowel fistula
- Ureteric injury
- Bladder injury
- Injury to blood vessels
- Stoma formation
- Issues with fertility
- Early menopause and long-term consequences due to that

Not all complications and injuries to organs are detected at the time of surgery. Close follow-up of these patients is done in the tertiary centre.

Rectovaginal Endometriosis

Deep endometriosis in the posterior pelvis frequently affects the space between the anterior wall of the rectosigmoid and the posterior vaginal wall and is usually referred to as rectovaginal endometriosis. The most consistent symptom differentiating it from the pain associated with less severe and other forms of endometriosis or adenomyosis is pain on intercourse or dyspareunia. In addition, in the more severe groups, pain on defecation is a common symptom due to the proximity to, or invasion of, the bowel.

There is limited evidence supporting the sustained effectiveness and acceptability of medical therapies in improving the symptoms of rectovaginal endometriosis (4–6). Consequently, surgical treatment has been proposed to completely excise the deep rectovaginal disease (7–9).

Advances in instrumentation and surgical experience have led to laparoscopic treatment superseding alternative surgical routes such as laparotomy and transvaginal excision. It is well-recognized that surgery for deep endometriosis with bowel involvement is complex and can be associated with serious and potentially life-threatening complications (10). For these reasons, the European Society of Human Reproduction and Embryology (ESHRE) Guidelines on the "Management of Women with Endometriosis" recommend that clinicians refer women with suspected or diagnosed deep endometriosis to a centre of expertise that offers all available treatments in a multidisciplinary context (11).

In 2006, the British Society for Gynaecological Endoscopy (BSGE) developed specialist endometriosis centres (Endocentres), where patients could be treated by surgeons who work in multidisciplinary teams, audit their outcomes and perform sufficient workload to maintain their surgical skills (12). This type of surgery requires enhanced laparoscopic skills, primarily because of the need to overcome distorted anatomy and operate in proximity to delicate gastrointestinal, genitourinary and vascular structures (13).

In view of the paucity of world literature data pertaining to the effectiveness and safety of this highly complex surgery for a common gynaecological condition, a prospective, multicentre cohort study was done in 2018 (13) to estimate the effectiveness of surgery on patient-reported symptoms associated with endometriosis as well as its impact on women's health-related QoL and safety by examining rates of surgical complications using data collected from the BSGE Endocentres dataset. The outcomes were assessed in both the short term (at 6 months) and longer term (at 2 years) following surgery.

"Laparoscopic Excision of Deep Rectovaginal Endometriosis in BSGE Endometriosis Centres: A Multicentre Prospective Cohort Study" was the largest study of its kind in the world. Using data from the endometriosis centres, the study looked at nearly 5,000 patients who had surgery for severe endometriosis, performed by more than 100 different surgeons in 51 different hospitals (13).

All types of pain symptoms improved: Premenstrual pain, menstrual pain, non-cyclical pain, back pain, pain with sexual intercourse and pain on voiding and on opening the bowels. A significant reduction in the need for analgesia supported the findings of an overall reduction in pain symptoms. Bowel symptoms including frequency, urgency, incomplete emptying and constipation also improved.

The conclusion was that laparoscopic surgical excision of rectovaginal endometriosis appears to be effective in treating pelvic pain and bowel symptoms and improving health-related quality of life and has a low rate of serious perioperative and late complications when performed in recognized specialist centres (13).

Thoracic Endometriosis

Thoracic endometriosis is where endometrial tissue is located in the chest cavity. It may be on the diaphragm or the lungs.

Symptoms of thoracic endometriosis include chest pain, shortness of breath, coughing up blood or recurrent collapsed lung. CT scan or an MRI scan is the diagnostic tool for thoracic endometriosis.

Video-assisted laparoscopy (VL) and video-assisted thoracoscopic surgery (VATS) are usually used to view the suspected endometriosis tissue.

The management of this can only be provided in a tertiary centre. Endometriosis tissue in the thoracic cavity can be removed using minimally invasive video-assisted thoracoscopic surgery (VATS) or robotically, in selected cases. Endometriosis can also involve the diaphragm, which may need to be repaired minimally invasively. A team of a consultant thoracic surgeon and gynaecologists work together to treat both pelvic and thoracic endometriosis in a single procedure or in staged procedures.

Follow-up of patients in a Specialist Endometriosis Centre: Each patient is usually seen by the endometriosis specialist nurse after 2–4 weeks and reviewed in the clinic by the specialist gynaecologist in 3 months. Follow-up continues for 12 months to 2 years depending on the type of the surgery.

FUTURE CHALLENGES

In the future, one of the challenges will be to decide how far or how wide the scope of the Specialist Endometriosis Centre should be. There has been a great deal of international interest in developing centres.

Women suffer with chronic pain and psychological symptoms that impair their QoL. Health services and the wider economy suffer through utilization of substantial health care resources and restrictions placed on women's physical functioning that can lead to absenteeism and the inability to fulfil domestic and professional duties (14).

Future studies should consider randomizing between laparoscopic surgery and non-surgical therapy or alternatively compare different laparoscopic surgical interventions. The morbidity associated with rectovaginal endometriosis has a substantial economic impact due to the related reduction in activity both socially and in the workplace. Thus, any future studies should include formal economic analysis to weigh the costs of surgical management against clinical, health service and societal gains (13).

KEY POINT SUMMARY

- The Specialist Endometriosis Centre has a team consisting of gynaecologists with expertise in diagnosing and managing endometriosis including advanced laparoscopic surgical skills, pain specialists, radiologists, urologists, colorectal surgeons, thorax surgeons and psychologists.
- The Specialist Endometriosis Centre closely collaborates with its IVF clinic, offering advanced fertility treatments including oocyte donation and gestational surrogacy.
- Laparoscopic surgical excision of rectovaginal endometriosis appears to be effective in treating pelvic pain and bowel symptoms and improving health-related quality of life and has a low rate of major complications when performed in specialist centres.

As a GP, you must know the nearest Specialist Endometriosis Centre in your area.

REFERENCES

1. D'Hooghe T, Hummelshoj L. Multi-disciplinary centres/networks of excellence for endometriosis management and research: A proposal. *Hum Reprod* 2006;21:2743–8.
2. Saridogan E, Byrne D. The British Society for Gynaecological Endoscopy endometriosis centres project. *Gynecol Obstet Invest* 2013;76:10–3. doi:10.1159/000348520
3. de Kok L, van Hanegem N, van Kesteren P, et al. Endometriosis centers of expertise in the Netherlands: Development toward regional networks of multidisciplinary care. *Health Sci Rep* 2022;5:e447. doi:10.1002/hsr2.447
4. Vercellini P, Crosignani PG, Somigliana E, et al. Medical treatment for rectovaginal endometriosis: What is the evidence? *Hum Reprod* 2009;24:2504–14.

5. Fedele L, Bianchi S, Zanconato G, et al. Gonadotropin-releasing hormone agonist treatment for endometriosis of the rectovaginal septum. *Am J Obstet Gynecol* 2000;183:1462–7.
6. Busacca M, Somigliana E, Bianchi S, et al. Post-operative GnRH analogue treatment after conservative surgery for symptomatic endometriosis stage III–IV: A randomized controlled trial. *Hum Reprod* 2001;16:2399–402.
7. Jerby BL, Kessler H, Falcone T, et al. Laparoscopic management of colorectal endometriosis. *Surg Endosc* 1999;13:1125–8.
8. Redwine DB. Laparoscopic en bloc resection for treatment of the obliterated cul-de-sac in endometriosis. *J Reprod Med* 1992;37:695–8.
9. Emmanuel KR, Davis C. Outcomes and treatment options in rectovaginal endometriosis. *Curr Opin Obstet Gynecol* 2005;17:399–402.
10. Meuleman C, Tomassetti C, D'Hoore A, et al. Surgical treatment of deeply infiltrating endometriosis with colorectal involvement. *Hum Reprod Update* 2011;17:311–26.
11. Dunselman GA, Vermeulen N, Becker C, et al. ESHRE guideline: Management of women with endometriosis. *Hum Reprod* 2014;29:400–12.
12. Saridogan E, Byrne D. The British Society for Gynaecological Endoscopy endometriosis centres project. *Gynecol Obstet Invest* 2013;76:10–13.
13. Byrne D, Curnow T, Smith P, et al. On behalf of BSGE Endometriosis Centres. Laparoscopic excision of deep rectovaginal endometriosis in BSGE endometriosis centres: A multicentre prospective cohort study. *BMJ open* 2018;8:e018924. doi:10.1136/bmjopen-2017-018924
14. Soliman AM, Yang H, Du EX, et al. The direct and indirect costs associated with endometriosis: A systematic literature review. *Hum Reprod* 2016;31:712–22.

FURTHER READING

American Association of Gynaecological Laparoscopists. www.aagl.org
American Society of Reproductive Medicine. www.asrm.org
British Society for Gynaecological Endoscopy. www.bsge.org.uk
Endometriosis: Diagnosis and management. NICE Guideline (NG73). 2017 Sep 6. www.nice.org.uk
Endometriosis UK. www.endometriosis-uk.org
European Society of Human Reproduction and Embryology. www.eshre.eu
NHS Inform—Endometriosis
Royal College of Obstetricians and Gynaecologists. www.rcog.org.uk

CHAPTER 12

Delayed Diagnosis: How to Reduce the Risks

....

Failure to diagnose endometriosis or a delay in diagnosis is not necessarily negligent, but a claimant may have a case if they can demonstrate that a doctor's management fell below the expected standard. For example, by not adequately examining the patient or by not considering the diagnosis when a patient presents with those signs and symptoms as described in the NICE Guidance.

Internationally, women face significant barriers and times to diagnosis. The prolonged time without a diagnosis may result in treatment delay, with clinical implications of chronic pain and an unknown effect on fertility outcomes.

As delays in diagnosis extend, those suffering from endometriosis incur more cost and frequently experience a reduction in quality of life.

An All-Party Parliamentary Group (APPG) survey was undertaken prior to the onset of the pandemic and lockdown. Survey ran from 10 February 2020 until 24 March 2020, and 13,000 responses were received, including 10,783 responses eligible for this report.

THE APPG ON ENDOMETRIOSIS FINDINGS: 2020

Sir David Amess MP, Chair of the APPG on Endometriosis, says:

> *The report provides a stark picture of the reality of living with endometriosis, including the huge, life-long impact it may have on all aspects of life. It is not acceptable that endometriosis and its potentially debilitating and damaging symptoms are often ignored or not*

DOI: 10.1201/9781032684819-14

taken seriously—or downplayed as linked to the menstrual cycle and periods. All UK Governments must take the recommendations in this report seriously and act to ensure that everyone with endometriosis has a prompt diagnosis, along with access to the physical and mental health support they need to manage their condition.

Our report highlights the urgent need for more research into the experiences and needs of those from LGBTQ+, black, Asian and minority ethnic backgrounds. We must do more to understand the health inequalities and barriers for those from minority backgrounds in accessing the care they need.

The APPG will not rest until tangible improvements are delivered to all those who suffer from this condition:

- 81% said endometriosis has impacted their mental health negatively or very negatively, and 90% would have liked access to psychological support but were not offered this
- Over 60% of respondents were seen in hospital settings where there is not necessarily the expertise to operate on or treat them effectively. NICE Guideline [NG73] on *Endometriosis: Diagnosis and management* (2017) set out the NHS baseline for endometriosis care. Despite being adopted by the NHS in each nation of the UK, the NICE Guideline has not been implemented (1)
- Only 19% knew if they had been seen in an endometriosis specialist centre, yet 84% of respondents reported bowel symptoms due to endometriosis All those with suspected or confirmed deep endometriosis, for example, involving the bowel, should be seen in an endometriosis specialist centre where there are the necessary skills and expertise from multidisciplinary teams to treat these patients
- Many with endometriosis felt that they are being failed by the system, and even when they have a diagnosis, they were unable to access the care they need—54% were not very or not at all confident they could get an appointment with a gynaecologist about their endometriosis symptoms if they felt they needed to (pre-COVID-19)

Diagnosis

- It takes 8 years on average from onset of symptoms to receiving a diagnosis, the same length of time as it did a decade ago
- Prior to receiving a diagnosis of endometriosis, due to their symptoms:

    ○ 58% visited the GP over 10 times
    ○ 21% visited doctors in hospital 10 times or more

- ○ 53% went to A&E
- ○ 27% went to A&E three or more times
- The APPG also acknowledges that not everyone who lives with endometriosis will identify as female

Access to Treatments

- 26% found their GP(s) helpful or very helpful, whilst 46% found their GP(s) unhelpful or very unhelpful
- 43% found their gynaecologist(s) helpful or very helpful, whilst 32% found their gynaecologist(s) unhelpful or very unhelpful
- 54% were not very or not at all confident they could get an appointment with a gynaecologist about their endometriosis symptoms if they felt they needed to
- Only 19% knew if they were seen in an endometriosis specialist centre
- 58% would have liked fertility support and treatment but were not offered it despite endometriosis doubling the risk of infertility in under 35s (2)
- 72% were not given any written information when diagnosed, leaving them without the knowledge and advice they need to make informed choices about their health care

Impact

As well as the physical impact, the survey demonstrated the impact endometriosis and its symptoms can have on all aspects of life including education, career, relationships, social life and mental health:

- 95% said that endometriosis/the symptoms of endometriosis had impacted their wellbeing negatively or very negatively
- 90% would have liked access to psychological support but were not offered this
- 89% felt isolated due to their endometriosis
- 81% said endometriosis has impacted their mental health negatively or very negatively
- 42% said they often, or very often, had time off school because of endometriosis symptoms, with 12% missing exams at school often or very often
- 38% were concerned about losing their job, whilst 35% had a reduced income due to endometriosis

Recommendations

- It is vital for health care practitioners to recognize the symptoms of endometriosis to be able to support diagnosis and ongoing treatment and care
- Awareness and education with the public are needed of what a "normal" period is, the symptoms of endometriosis and other menstrual conditions and when to seek help

Reducing Time for Diagnosis

- Currently, diagnosis time is an average of 8 years—the same as it was a decade ago. The APPG is seeking a commitment from governments in all four nations to reduce average diagnosis times with targets of 4 years or less by 2025, and a year or less by 2030
- Building NHS capacity to appropriately diagnose those with endometriosis
- That the UK governments ensure the NICE Guideline and Quality Standards on Endometriosis are implemented
- Prompt referrals from primary to secondary care, including for diagnostic laparoscopy, by ensuring capacity within gynaecology departments and specialist centres for endometriosis
- Identify learning from the Rapid Diagnostic Centres being implemented to reduce times for diagnosing endometriosis
- All areas to have a managed clinical network to coordinate endometriosis care
- All patients with confirmed or suspected endometriosis should have access to a gynaecologist with expertise in diagnosing and managing endometriosis, including skills in laparoscopic surgery
- Rather than relying on strong prescription painkillers or strong opioid drugs, which is not the only option, other interventions, such as pelvic physiotherapy, can be accessed
- Access to fertility services should be available to those with endometriosis who require them
- Despite up to 10% of those with the disease having endometriosis outside the pelvic cavity, the NICE Guideline covers only endometriosis within the pelvic cavity. Pathways need to be established for non-pelvic endometriosis starting with thoracic endometriosis
- These should be included in an updated NICE Guideline covering all types of endometrioses
- Investment in research to discover the cause of the disease, better treatment, management options and, one day, a cure

- Ensure that psychological support becomes a part of person's treatment plan
- Provide patient information, so patients are not left in the dark about their disease
- The APPG calls for NICE to reconsider the decision not to support the use of Visanne, or Dienogest, by the NHS. Visanne is used to treat endometriosis pelvic pain and is widely available in the rest of the world including Europe and Australia
- The APPG would like to see menstrual wellbeing included as compulsory in the school curriculums across the UK, as it now is in England, to overcome the taboo of talking about periods and ensure all adolescents understand what a normal period is and when to seek help

Fertility

- There is a need to look holistically at the individual including their desires or concerns around fertility
- NICE Guidelines: Fertility problems, assessment and treatment (CG156) should be followed including early referral to specialist
- If an individual's endometriosis or the treatments they are receiving could impact their fertility, they should have access to NHS treatment for fertility preservation

Work and Benefits

- Ensure those with endometriosis who need it have statutory support and don't face discrimination due to lack of understanding and societal taboos around menstrual conditions. This includes access to PIP and other disability allowances—ensuring guidance around endometriosis and its potential impact on work is clear to those assessing applications
- Ensure those with the disease who need it have access to statutory sick pay (SSP)
- Endometriosis should not be a taboo subject, and organizations and the UK governments should adopt an open culture when it comes to talking about menstrual health
- The UK governments should lead by example in encouraging employers to become "Endometriosis Friendly"

Mental Health

- Integrated mental health support as part of the endometriosis pathway
- Updating the NICE Guideline on Endometriosis to ensure mental health support is provided to patients who need it

- Ensuring the NICE Guideline is followed so that patients are not waiting on average 8 years for a diagnosis potentially, leaving patients with long-term mental health issues

Education

- Devolved administrations to ensure menstrual wellbeing education is mandatory in all schools
- Ensure all young people across the UK have access to the same level of menstrual wellbeing education
- In England, the government needs to ensure new education on menstrual wellbeing is implemented in all schools, and teachers are given sufficient support and resources

Diversity and Inclusion

- Recognition that more needs to be done to ensure inclusivity and equality of access to endometriosis services
- Governments to work with the NHS to ensure nobody faces additional barriers in accessing health care due to their race, gender, sexuality, ability or social status and ensure that those with additional needs such as learning disabilities have access to appropriate patient information and resources
- Address health disparities for Black, Asian and minority people with endometriosis
- End the gender and ethnicity data gaps in research for those from Black, Asian and minority ethnic groups backgrounds
- As identified in the NICE Quality Standards, those who don't identify as female may find it distressing to attend appointments in a women's hospital or dedicated women's unit and may need to be seen in another clinic or setting in line with their individual preference
- Where possible, non-gendered language should be used by health care practitioners in relation to endometriosis and other gynaecological conditions
- Training should be provided by RCGP and RCOG for HCPs in providing care and support for those with gynaecological conditions who do not identify as female
- For those with pre-existing mental health conditions or disabilities (learning or otherwise), there may be additional barriers in accessing care
- Evidence should be gathered into the barriers faced by those with additional needs and ensure their additional needs are met

WHO RESPONSE ABOUT ADDRESSING
CURRENT CHALLENGES AND PRIORITIES

WHO aims to stimulate and support the adoption of effective policies and interventions to address endometriosis globally, especially in low- and middle-income countries and is partnering with multiple stakeholders, including academic institutions and other organizations that are actively involved in research, to identify effective models of prevention, diagnosis, treatment and care of endometriosis.

According to WHO, the following are the priorities related to endometriosis:

- Raising awareness about endometriosis among health care providers, women, men, adolescents, teachers and wider communities. Local, national and international information campaigns to educate the public and health care providers about normal and abnormal menstrual health and symptoms are needed

- Training all health care providers to improve their competency and skills to screen, diagnose, manage or refer patients with endometriosis. This can range from basic training of primary health care providers to recognize endometriosis, to the advanced training of specialist surgeons and multidisciplinary teams

- Ensuring that primary health care plays a role in screening, identifying and providing basic pain management of endometriosis, in situations where gynaecologists or advanced multidisciplinary specialists are unavailable

- Advocating for health policies that ensure access to at least a minimum level of treatment and support for patients with endometriosis.

- Setting up referral systems and care pathways consisting of well-linked primary health care centres and secondary and tertiary centres with advanced imaging, pharmacologic, surgical, fertility and multidisciplinary interventions

- Strengthening capacity of health systems to achieve early diagnosis and management of endometriosis by enhancing availability of equipment (e.g., ultrasound or magnetic resonance imaging) and pharmaceuticals (e.g., nonsteroidal analgesics, combined oral contraceptives and progestin-based contraceptives)

- Increasing research on the pathogenesis, pathophysiology, natural progression, genetic and environmental risk factors, prognosis, disease classification, non-invasive diagnostic biomarkers, personalized treatments and other treatment paradigms, role of surgery, novel targeted therapeutics, curative therapies and preventive interventions in endometriosis (3,4)

- Accelerating collaborative global action to improve access to reproductive health care for women globally, including in low- and middle-income countries

MEDICAL DEFENCE UNION (MDU) CASES

During 2020 and 2021, there were 32 incidents reported to the MDU involving endometriosis. A common factor in these incidents involved a complaint or claim following an allegation of a missed or delayed diagnosis (5).

A delayed diagnosis can lead to prolonged pain and suffering and may cause other physical and psychological problems for the patient, such as infertility, anxiety and depression. Some of the findings from the incidents are listed following:

- The alleged delay in diagnosis from the time the patient presented ranged from 4 months to nearly 5 years
- The age ranges of the patients diagnosed with endometriosis ranged from 15 to 51 years
- Three-quarters of the incidents (24) were related to complaints and a quarter (8) to claims for compensation. Of the complaint files, two later became a claim for clinical negligence. No cases were referred to the Health Service Ombudsman or GMC
- Three-quarters of complaint files related to patients who were seen in general practice, all having been seen by a GP
- Of the eight claims files, three related to care provided by a GP and five related to care provided by obstetrics and gynaecology. Of the latter, two related to private care rather than that provided by the NHS

How to Reduce the Risk of Delayed Diagnosis

- If a telephone consultation relates to abdominal pain, pain that is worse during periods, painful sexual intercourse, inability to get pregnant or cyclical bowel or bladder symptoms, make sure you appoint the patient for face-to-face examination
- Make sure all relevant symptoms are clearly documented including the detailed history, patient's concerns and abdominal and pelvic examination
- Do discuss with the patient differential diagnosis, management plan and follow-up plan and document in the notes

- Take into account patient's family history of gynaecological problems including endometriosis. Some research suggests that there may be a genetic element to the condition and some families may be more susceptible than others
- Involve the patient in decision-making of management plan and document in the notes
- Ensure an appropriate timely referral for further treatment or procedure is done
- When a referral is made, make sure there is a system in place to check that an appointment follows so that she is not lost in the system
- The practice should have a safe system for following up of abnormal results including pelvic ultrasound scan
- Give advice to make an early appointment if pain gets worse and document in notes for staff to read and understand
- Do an educational event in-house about diagnosis and referral pathway for endometriosis and include that in your professional development plan (PDP)
- Ensure your practice has a robust system of significant event, learning event, analyzing patient care and safety and distribution to all members of the team
- Provide patients with an explanation and apology if something does go wrong, particularly if the outcome is poor or unexpected. Take steps to deal with the consequences and arrange appropriate treatment and follow-up. Contact MPS/MDU at the earliest opportunity if you have any concerns

KEY POINT SUMMARY

- Remote consultations can result in delayed diagnosis.
- Varied non-specific symptoms, normal pelvic scan, clinician's non-awareness of symptoms and poor access to specialist services are resulting in delay in diagnosis.
- Face-to-face appointment involving the patient in decision-making of management plan, proper documentation in the notes and timely referral to specialist endometriosis consultant can reduce the risk of delayed diagnosis.

REFERENCES

1. NICE. *Endometriosis: Diagnosis and management.* NICE Guidelines (NG 73). NICE. 2017. www.nice.org.uk/guidance/ng73 (accessed 11 Nov 2024).
2. Prescott J, Farland LV, Tobias DK, et al. A prospective cohort study of endometriosis and subsequent risk of infertility. *Hum Reprod* 2016;31(7):1475–82.

3. Zondervan KT, Becker CM, Missmer SA. Endometriosis. *N Engl J Med* 2020;382:1244–56.
4. Horne AW, Saunders PTK, Abokhrais IM, et al. Top ten endometriosis research priorities in the UK-and Ireland. *Lancet* 2017;389:2191–92.
5. Avoiding Diagnosis Delays in Endometriosis. *Diagnostic delays for endometriosis can occur, with many of the symptoms similar to other common medical conditions.* MDU. 2022 Mar 7.

FURTHER READING

All Party Parliamentary Group on Endometriosis, Endometriosis UK. *Endometriosis in the UK: Time for change.* London: Endometriosis UK, 2020. www.endometriosis-uk.org/sites/default/files/files/Endometriosis%20APPG%20Report%20Oct%202020.pdf
NICE. *Endometriosis: Diagnosis and management.* NICE Guideline 73. NICE. 2017. www.nice.org.uk/ng73

CHAPTER 13

Living with Endometriosis: Stories from Patients and Their Families

....

Lucy Bowker's Story

....

Lucy Bowker and Tony Bowker

DESPERATE PLEA TO DOCTORS FROM AN OLDHAM NURSE WHO SUFFERS WITH ENDOMETRIOSIS TO UNDERSTAND THIS CONDITION BETTER

Despite the prevalence and the severity of the condition, there remain many challenges in endometriosis care, with significant time to diagnosis, a lack of patient-friendly diagnostics and a need for more targeted treatments.

I first began experiencing symptoms of endometriosis when my periods started, around 12 years ago. I would always have painful periods and heavy bleeding and occasionally had to miss school. I just thought that this was normal, and everyone's period was like mine. When I was growing up, I had a lot of male friends, and it wasn't something that I felt that I could talk to anyone else about.

As the years went on, throughout being a teenager, the period pain would get worse. I would visit the GP countless times complaining about this. During this time, it was never suggested to me that anything could be wrong, and I felt my concerns were not listened to or valid. I started the contraceptive pill around age 14/15 as the GP advised me that it would manage how heavy my periods were and help with the pain. It did seem to help me somewhat, and I remained on the contraceptive pill for 3–4 years. Looking back now, I know this to be that this simply masked my symptoms and did not treat them. The contraceptive pill does not prevent spread or growth of endometriosis.

At 18, I got pregnant (despite being on the contraceptive pill) and had a healthy baby boy. Following giving birth, I experienced an extended

DOI: 10.1201/9781032684819-16

period of bleeding. Unfortunately, this persisted for 9 months for me despite being prescribed various contraceptive pills, injections—you name it, I had it. It was for this reason I believe that the GP finally listened to me and referred me to gynaecology. For a lot of people, it can take a long time and certainly a lot longer than I had to wait.

I was seen quite soon after by gynaecology at a local health centre. The consultant told me that I could not have endometriosis as I was so young and tried to manage my symptoms with various medications which did not help. One of the medications he prescribed was tranexamic acid, which is used to reduce the amount of bleeding, but this had no effect, and at this stage, I was changing a maternity pad up to 10 times a day. I could not believe that the consultant deemed this to be normal.

After numerous appointments over the next 10 months or so, I was listed for surgery, which was carried out at a private hospital as an NHS patient. The surgery I had was an exploratory laparoscopy during which I was told they had found "mild endometriosis." Following this diagnosis, I was referred to my local hospital under the care of the gynaecologists.

Whilst I did not appreciate it at the time, the doctors I saw at the hospital were not specialists in endometriosis and their main practice was not endometriosis. My management at this time consisted almost solely of pain relief.

I did, however, see the endometriosis link nurse who discussed with me the various symptoms I was experiencing including painful sex. She seemed to think that my problems were not necessarily endometriosis, but this was later confirmed to be endometriosis. She instead prescribed the use of dilators and suggested that my pain was more connected to anxiety in the context of me expecting the sex to hurt—there was no psychological support provided at all.

After a few appointments and persisting failures of contraceptive attempts to control my symptoms, I was offered a course of Prostap. I was told at the time that by receiving Prostap, during the time I was receiving treatment, I would be in an artificial menopause and should not experience symptoms of endometriosis. The endometriosis should not be able to grow, and I should be able to live a "normal life."

The side effects of Prostap are that of menopause but I, as do the majority of women with endometriosis, thought those to be reasonable when you consider the alternative. My life at this point was littered with hospital attendances. I would be treated in A&E and receive strong painkillers before being sent up to the ward for "pain management," which consisted of a junior doctor reviewing me and prescribing another medication which inevitably would not work. During this time, I was training to be a nurse and balancing this with caring for my son (by this point, age 2).

Whilst I was on Prostap my symptoms reduced significantly, and I felt optimistic for the first time in a long time. I could engage with my hobbies, work and study and spend better time with my family.

However, this was not going to last as you cannot take Prostap indefinitely. As with the menopause, the risks include that of osteoporosis, and although I was taking hormone replacement therapy, a DEXA scan (bone density scan) showed that my bones were not quite as dense as they might have wanted them to be, and they suggested that I take a break from Prostap.

I came off Prostap, and my symptoms returned with a vengeance. They typically recommend that you have at least 6 months between courses of Prostap, which I almost managed. During the time that I was recovering from the Prostap, the endometriosis was allowed to spread.

In November 2019, I was admitted to hospital with abdominal pain and sent to the gynaecology ward. Despite my history, the doctors thought that I may have appendicitis and took me to theatre for appendectomy. This was carried out, but following surgery, I was seen by the hospital's endometriosis specialist (and specialist nurse) who requested that my onward care be with her rather than the other gynaecology consultants at the hospital.

I resumed Prostap in early 2020, and this time remained on the drug until I had my next endometriosis surgery in June 2021.

Prior to surgery, I had an MRI scan that revealed that my uterus was adhered to my bowel, and it required separating.

I had the surgery carried out in June 2021, and my recovery from surgery was unfortunately complicated. My wounds would not heal, and I had persisting infection which required two more operations, the last of which being in October 2021.

During this time, I did, however, get relief from the endometriosis symptoms, but that was relatively short-lived, and my symptoms returned around January 2022. I had an MRI scan at this time to assess the extent of my endometriosis.

During this time, I transferred my care to a more specialist hospital as I was showing signs of quite widespread DIE (deep infiltrative endometriosis). In March 2022, I found out that I was pregnant with a baby that we have been trying for since approximately 2020.

In April 2022, we received news that our baby was not one but two. Unfortunately, the second baby was in my left fallopian tube and required removing. Despite this, baby #1 was still healthy.

Shortly after the surgery to remove the second baby in April 2022, I began bleeding quite heavily. I had numerous scans which confirmed that my baby was healthy, but around mid-May 2022, we found out that there was a subchorionic haemorrhage next to him that was growing. At our 12-week appointment, we also received the news that our baby required further investigation as they were showing signs suggestive of a developmental problem.

We underwent further screening which thankfully confirmed that everything was normal and inadvertently confirmed with us that he was a boy!

Despite the good news, I continued to bleed heavily, and I changed my pad numerous times a day which were soaked with blood. One day in particular, I changed my pad 22 times, so I went to the hospital. They were concerned, so I was kept in hospital for a few nights before being discharged.

I remained home for little under a day before reattending. Whilst in hospital, I had a large antepartum haemorrhage and lost 4 L of blood. We had to make the difficult decision to compassionately induce our baby despite him being 17 weeks gestated. The doctor put it plainly to me that if I did not take this course of action, I would die and then neither of us would live. I delivered my baby, and we named him Euan Thomas.

Following discharge, I continued to feel unwell. It became apparent that I had retained part of my placenta, and I had to return to hospital for it to be surgically removed. Throughout this time, I feel as though I did get the emotional support that I needed in regard to bereavement and losing my son. However, the support for living with a long-term chronic condition and how it affects the rest of your life is non-existent.

In July 2022, I had an appointment with the endometriosis specialists, and they advised me that my MRI taken in January 2022 revealed that the endometriosis had spread to my bowel, my ureters, my bladder and my ligaments in my pelvis.

The only options were for extensive surgery to try and preserve my fertility or to carry out a hysterectomy.

I opted for fertility-sparing surgery, and I was referred to be discussed in the gynaecology MDT.

Whilst waiting for surgery, my condition has progressed further, and I now have endometriosis on my belly button and abdominal wall.

I am now unable to urinate without a catheter, I bleed from my belly button whenever I menstruate, and I am on long-term steroids as my body no longer produces cortisol.

The endometriosis diagnosis per se did not change my life but rather confirmed something within me that I always knew deep down. A diagnosis is not a magic label that makes things better, but it does allow you access to treatment options that may not be open to people who do not have a formal diagnosis.

Endometriosis is now encompassing almost every aspect of my life. I am currently in hospital more often than I am not. The endometriosis causes me immense pain and prevents me from working as often as I want to; the impact of the endometriosis on my medical health is quite separate to the effect it has on your mental health. I am not able to engage in activities that a typical 24-year-old would. I am now in a position whereby I must take a medication just so my body doesn't give up on me because it does not generate its own cortisol. This is something that until it happened, I never thought could arise from something that was explained to me at an early age as "just a bad period."

SUMMARY POINTS BY DR ANITA SHARMA

- An example of women being treated like second-class citizens.
- If this were a condition that resulted in men enduring agony, time lost from work, plans cancelled constantly and people constantly questioning your pain, I am sure treatment would be better and even a cure forthcoming.
- The fact that she is a nurse means there will be somebody on the front line, batting for women with endometriosis and countering the prejudice against those with the condition.

ENDO AND MY FAMILY: A FATHER'S STORY

Tony Bowker

Endometriosis has been a part of my life for well over a decade. Both my daughters suffer with this terrible disease, which has, at times, devastated us and taken away a childhood which should have been full of joy, fun and wonder.

From the age of 11–12 years, my daughter had started her periods as any other child of the same sex and age; however, she had indicated to her mum that the pain she felt and heavy periods she was having didn't seem the same as they should be, but mum reassured her not to worry as this would get better with time.

As a father, these things were something I wasn't made aware of as they were women's problems and hugely private things and something you don't really share with your dad or any male friends or your family, so I was not aware of what was happening privately.

I did know that she was having issues but didn't realize the extent of her issues, and as she had attended doctors' appointments at the time, my wife made me more aware of what they thought and what the next step would be to help her to elevate the pain and suffering. But as we found for a long time, we would be fobbed off and told basically to get on with it as this was normal for a child of her age to suffer like she was.

Time passed by and my daughter was in high school and at times really struggled with her understanding of her situation, which was only matched by her tutors who couldn't understand or even care about her situation. Over time, her education was interrupted with absences and avoidance of lessons such as physical education and sheer embarrassment at her blood loss at the worst and most inconvenient times.

Eventually, doctors did listen to us, and referrals went in to finally get further medical investigations underway. I had learned and understood more about what had been happening to her over the years, and my hidden fears, worries and concerns would be answered. Unfortunately the ultrasound didn't show anything of note, and the opportunity to diagnose what we now know was gone and the long process began again.

Her struggles continued for a long time to come. Further appointments and days off school led to me or my wife having to take time out of work to care for her or to attend further appointments or take her to A&E at 3 a.m. in the morning, leading to her being admitted and spending days and weeks on a ward in gynae or another observation ward where again she was dealt with by inexperienced doctors and staff who did not know what they were dealing with.

You can only use the same words or reassurance with someone before even what you say to your child becomes like a broken record, and you start to stop believing yourself. Over time, we had been in most of the hospitals in our local area of Manchester, spending so much time that we were worried about her education. After all, our daughter had aspirations of becoming a nurse or a professional athlete, and all of this was breaking her belief.

Eventually and after years of frustrations, she was granted a laparoscopy, which would diagnose endometriosis was present. This was the cause of all her issues and upset on us all. We were going to finally get her life on track. Unfortunately, this wouldn't be the case, and after many operations that were to come to take the endo away only for it to keep returning, we found that this was to be a problem that will possibly continue for the rest of her life. The scars on her body are permanent reminders of what she has gone through.

I know what she has had to face, and as I write this brief summary, I can reflect on my personal journey, and I immediately feel the same pain and upset and uselessness I've felt for so many years. This horrible unfair disease has taken so much away from us—her chances of becoming a mum herself and giving us grandchildren almost taken away. She is, these days, struggling with the same pain, and her bladder is no longer working and she is permanently catheterized. She had to take so much time off from work, and she's been clinging on hoping for an answer. There is always hope and the belief that a cure will be found, but this seems to be so far away. For me, now, my second daughter is suffering with the same problems, and the struggle continues. She has recently undergone a laparoscopy, and we are awaiting the results and the same journey begins. This has affected me as a parent. I know too much about this that I feel scared, but I do use the experience and knowledge to educate others who have children going through the same issues.

Siobhan Kennett's Story

....

Siobhan Kennett and James Kennett

I first heard the word "endometriosis" back in January 2023 from my GP, and I had my first surgery to officially confirm the diagnosis and removal of endometriosis in October 2023 at the age of 31.

Prior to this, I had been experiencing symptoms of endometriosis for almost 10 years, and over time, the symptoms were getting worse—more frequent debilitating pain and I was unable to continue with normal activities.

Within that time, I've lost count of how many times I visited my GP complaining endlessly about chronic symptoms of feeling tired, fatigue, lack of energy, constipation, bloating, frequent urination and irregular periods.

Every time it was put down to mental health, stress, anxiety and depression. I was even told it was down to my job and shift work and that I should think about looking for new employment.

All I was offered for years was the contraceptive pill and antidepressants. I felt like I was being constantly fobbed off and not listened to, and I felt like the GP was not interested.

All the symptoms I was experiencing were always treated separately, and no one had ever thought to link them together or was even open to the possibility that they could all be related to the same problem.

So my endo journey started in August 2022, where I had gone back to my GP after experiencing months of irregular, painful periods and occasional spotting in between.

I knew within myself that something just wasn't quite right, and I was concerned that it was something else, other than what they had initially put down to "just stress." I even feared it could be cervical cancer.

DOI: 10.1201/9781032684819-17

I spoke with my GP and finally got an appointment for examination.

After my examination and not finding anything apparently wrong, referral was made for an internal ultrasound.

In September 2022, I had my first ultrasound and that indicated that I had cysts on my ovaries—which they told me were extremely common in women and should clear up by themselves in 3 months.

In January 2023, I went back and had my follow-up ultrasound—which no surprise to me showed the cysts were still there—because the symptoms I was experiencing had gotten worse.

Even though I had questions for the nurse who conducted the ultrasound, she was adamant that she wasn't allowed to answer them and that I should wait to speak to my GP. I left that clinic in tears.

Later that month, I spoke to my male GP who explained that with the symptoms I was experiencing and the "chocolate" cysts that were present on both of my ovaries indicated that I had endometriosis. But he admitted that he had no real knowledge of it, and I should use "credible Google sources" for more information while he put through a referral to a specialist gynaecologist.

I was left in a highly unstable, emotional state for 6 months. In July 2023, I saw a community gynaecologist.

She sat me down for a good hour and explained to me what endometriosis was. She made me feel normal about it, and with her, for the first time, I felt like I was being listened to.

She performed my third ultrasound and confirmed that I had endometriosis on my ovaries.

In August 2023, my husband and I decided to go private for care because of lengthy waiting time on the NHS of approximately 18 months to 2 years.

Both my husband and I, at the time, felt like we had no other option due to the amount of physical pain I was in and my deteriorating mental health other than to self-fund and go private.

By this point, my mental health had gotten so bad that I had frequent thoughts of suicide, unable to bear the idea of living another single day in this amount of physical pain.

At my initial consultation, I asked the private gynaecologist how severe my endometriosis was as no one had ever answered this question in spite of my repeated requests. He replied that because it was on both my ovaries, it did indicate a quite severe level of endometriosis. I then asked him, in his opinion, how long have I possibly had it for, and he replied probably for years.

He also explained to me that surgery is the only treatment option I have. He explained that during the procedure, he would remove the endometriosis on my ovaries and also remove any more endometriotic deposits.

So, in October 2023, I had my first laparoscopy and excision of endometriotic deposits.

I found out after speaking with my gynaecologist post-op that he found and removed an extensive amount of endo adhesions on my bladder, back of my vagina and beneath and in both of my ovaries. To the extent he said that my bladder was almost sandwiched to my ovaries.

That what I'd been experiencing for years was real and that all the symptoms weren't all just in my head.

That I wasn't just this this crazy, mentally ill, hormonal, hypochondriac woman that I'd been made out to be. Even, at times, left questioning my own health and sanity.

Experiencing endometriosis flare-ups is painfully crippling—they dictate what I wear, what I eat, how I feel, if I can go out and what I can do. It affects my social life and my relationship with my husband.

The disease is not only physically cruel and debilitating but also has a devastating emotional impact on your life and causes so much mental distress.

The whole ordeal has left me traumatized from being gaslighted for years. Overall, I feel like I have had such a negative experience with endometriosis.

PRESENT DAY 2024 AND SUMMARY POINTS TO CONCLUDE

I joined Endometriosis Awareness North this year.

I only wish I had known about them sooner; it would have made my journey with endo a lot easier, and I wouldn't have felt so alone. I have been left feeling so angry by my own experience of endo, and I wanted to turn that anger into something positive, and that is why I'm here helping them raise some much-needed awareness:

- I feel so strongly as a society how we view women, especially in regard to women's gynaecological and menstrual health. Things desperately need changing
- To remove and challenge the taboos and negative stigma that surround talking about women's health and normalize it
- To improve the overall treatment, diagnosis and quality of life of sufferers going forward
- To get the word "endometriosis" out there by raising awareness and get people talking about it

- To raise awareness that endo is not only a physical disease that affects the body but also has a devastating effect on the sufferers' mental health and impacts the individual's whole lifestyle and the relationships they have with others
- We need to end the relentless gaslighting women experience in regard to their health and health concerns
- And to ultimately put pressure on those in charge to make these positive changes in regard to women's health care

A HUSBAND'S STORY

James Kennett

My name is James, I'm 35 and husband to Siobhan. Just like Siobhan, I had never heard of the term "endometriosis" till it was mentioned to her by the doctor.

Living with this condition through Siobhan has not been easy, and it has changed the way we do things and even what we can do.

The earliest warning signs of this without knowing was about 5 years ago when we woke up early in the morning to go to work and Siobhan was bent over double in floods of tears complaining about crippling period pains.

It has been a hard and stressful journey together living with it, multiple visits to GP and battling to get a preliminary diagnosis.

Even after the surgical intervention, it has not cured her symptoms. We are told that it will return, and it is just a matter of when.

It has definitely taken a toll on both of us and the relationship not only physically but also emotionally and mentally. All I can do as a husband is to be there for her when she is experiencing the excruciating pain or mental strain.

It made me feel helpless to stand by and watch her experience such pain all the while wanting to take it away for her and knowing there was nothing I could physically do.

I also felt and shared the same frustrations as Siobhan. I saw her every time when she was gaslighted by GPs and practice nurses.

So much so, that when Siobhan was due to go in for her surgery, I myself experienced the mental toll of her condition and had to take 2 months sick leave from work for my own mental wellbeing due to stress and exhaustion to help take care of her both before and after her surgery, and I wouldn't have been able to have left her at home during her recovery and gone to work.

I'm thankful that after years of suffering with pain, one GP had finally taken her health concerns seriously and referred her for an initial internal ultrasound, and when Siobhan did go for her internal ultrasound investigations, the clinician found the cysts on her ovaries because otherwise it would have gone completely undetected.

There is one thing that I would say is to raise awareness of this condition among professionals and public. I strongly feel that as husbands/partners, we need to have a better understanding of this condition so that we can provide support to our wife/partner and sufferers at our workplace.

Courtney Ormrod's Story

....

Courtney Ormrod and Paul Ormrod

I was 12 years old when I first started to notice signs and symptoms of endometriosis. From my first period at school, I will never forget the amount of pain that struck me and literally stopped me in my tracks. The pain from just bleeding each month was horrifically excruciating, to the point I was throwing up and passing out from the pain.

I remember on many occasions having to crawl on my hands and knees to the bathroom to use the toilet and blacking out due to the extreme pain. I remember many times collapsing and being blue lighted to the hospital because I'd be screaming in pain due to the endometriosis growing and affecting my back horrifically, which prevented me being able to walk, stand or even move. I remember being in excruciating pain trying to use the toilet and blacking out, then choking on my sick and having to be put in the recovery position until I'd woken up.

Growing up not knowing what was wrong with my body was torturous. Constantly being told by health professionals and specialists that "the pain was most likely psychological" and "you are just hypersensitive to pain" pushed me to breaking point. A young girl constantly being dismissed, told she's basically crazy by the people you pray can help you the most is soul destroying.

I had to fight so hard to be believed when I came across the word "endometriosis," which a private physio informed me all about at the time and strongly believed I had this disease. If it wasn't for him, my fight would have taken even longer than the 7 years it took for my diagnosis. Seven years of pleading and trying to persuade professionals to listen to me, believe me and refer me to an endo specialist for a diagnostic surgery

DOI: 10.1201/9781032684819-18

was incredibly difficult. We are often told and in my case, "You're far too young to have endometriosis," "It's most likely IBS," "It's just bad periods and you have hypermobility, you'll grow out of it." It's just not acceptable, not acceptable to dismiss what a patient and young girl with obvious signs and symptoms of the disease is telling them.

I suffered and still do with crippling pains and symptoms that need to be listened to and taken more seriously. They are so important to be aware of, such as horrific contractions and cramping; heavy and prolonged bleeding with cycles and in-between; painful sexual intercourse; painful urinating and bowel movements; inability to pass urine; constipation and diarrhoea; nausea; fatigue; severe bloating; severe back, pelvic, leg and abdominal pain; painful digestion; upper abdominal, rib, shoulder and chest pains; joint pains; depression/low mood:

- My age was held against me
- Girls and women need to be listened to and taken seriously regardless of age and gender
- Women's health should be taken equally as seriously as men when they approach a GP or professional with health concerns
- My symptoms were not taken seriously by physicians including A&E
- If I was not seen privately by a physio and consultant in endometriosis specialist, it would have taken longer for my diagnosis
- I am fully committed to Endometriosis Awareness North raising awareness and promoting education among health care professionals

Endometriosis has greatly impacted my life. It left me unable to walk without crutches in my teens, in agonizing pain, missing out on socializing and hobbies and eventually left me bedridden, which caused my mental health to crumble. I missed out on my further education, unable to go to university and unable to chase my dreams of becoming a school teacher.

> By sharing my story, I hope to empower other women to get checked as soon as they can. I also urge women not to give up: Ask for a second opinion if you are not satisfied with the response.

A FATHER'S STORY

Paul Ormrod

Endometriosis renders parents impotent. Most parents intervene to help their child with an illness. Endometriosis is not like that. Before you know what it is, you are desperately looking for answers. You go down many false paths and take numerous wrong turns. Once you do know what it is, you are desperately seeking solutions.

However, with endometriosis, there are no final solutions. A laparoscopy may provide initial relief from some of the symptoms, but they always return. It's a heartbreaking journey for any parent to watch their daughter suffer from an early age into adulthood and not be able to do anything meaningful to help.

This impotence is exacerbated by the ignorance of the condition displayed by GPs and the NHS in general. The time taken to achieve a diagnosis demonstrates how poorly this disease is understood by professionals. As parents and carers, we suffer mentally alongside our child's own mental and physical suffering. There is no help available for those caring for an endometriosis sufferer just like the sufferers themselves. We, too, feel isolated and alone.

Other young girls and women and their families are busy getting on with their lives, and even though you explain the condition, you only receive platitudes. Even some members of your own family can't grasp the magnitude of this disease.

So as parents of an endometriosis sufferer, you feel isolated and cut off because you feel abandoned by the medical profession and the world in general.

Patient Stories: Summary from the Lead Author, Dr Anita Sharma

....

After reading these six stories my suggestion would be to have a learning event in your surgery.

Lead or Education GP to ask the following questions:

1. For patients presenting with painful periods, how often do you ask about painful sexual intercourse, rectal pain and pain during passing urine and defecation?
2. Does patient's age influence the clinical suspicion of endometriosis?
3. When would you consider referral to secondary care with suspected endometriosis?
4. Are you aware of referral to tertiary centres?

On the basis of the answers, you can organize an educational event in your practice with continuing professional development (CPD) points.

DOI: 10.1201/9781032684819-19

CHAPTER 14

Complications

....

Women with endometriosis can sometimes experience several complications.

Complications of untreated endometriosis depend on the site of the disease. Surgical or medical treatment of endometriosis, resulting in recurrence, complications during surgery and afterwards resulting in chronic pain, mental health issues and reduced quality of life are all well reported.

VARIOUS COMPLICATIONS

a. *Formation of adhesions*: Adhesions are when two or more organs are joined together with scar tissue. This complication arises when endometrial tissue causes bleeding in the pelvis. The bleeding leads to inflammation in the surrounding tissue and eventually the formation of scar tissue. Formation of adhesions caused by endometriosis or secondary to surgery can cause chronic pelvic pain, fertility problems and partial or complete bowel obstruction (1).

b. *Development of endometriomas*: These are ovarian cysts containing endometrium-like tissue and blood. Rupture of the endometrioma is a well-known complication and can affect fertility (2).

   They can be treated with surgery but may come back in the future if the endometriosis returns.

c. *Fertility problems*: Endometriosis is commonly associated with infertility, with a prevalence of 25–40% in infertile women compared with 0.5–5% in fertile women.

   It is unclear whether there is a causal link between endometriosis and infertility (2).

DOI: 10.1201/9781032684819-20

Complications related to severe endometriosis resulting in tubal adhesions, poor implantation and reduced ovarian reserve as well as reducing embryo quality (3–5) can lead to fertility problems. Even mild endometriosis can impair fertility (3).

Not all women with endometriosis will have problems with fertility, and some will eventually get pregnant without treatment.

Medication does not improve the fertility. Surgery to remove endometriotic deposits can sometimes help. In some women, IVF may be an option, but women with moderate to severe endometriosis tend to have a lower chance of getting pregnant with IVF than usual.

d. *Recurrence after treatment*: Endometriosis is a chronic disease, and prospective data indicate that recurrence after surgery ranges from 10–50% at 1 year and increases over time (6). Pain from endometriosis might become chronic even when visible disease has been removed.

A systematic review has shown that use of oral contraceptives can reduce pain after surgery and reduce recurrence of endometriomas and is as effective and better tolerated than gestrinone, mifepristone, or GnRH agonists without hypoestrogenic side effects (7). A randomized controlled trial has shown that the efficacy of the levonorgestrel-releasing intrauterine system (Mirena) is comparable with GnRH agonists in the relief of complications of chronic pelvic pain after surgery for endometriosis (8).

e. *Ectopic pregnancy*: An ectopic pregnancy occurs when a fertilized ovum implants and matures outside the uterine endometrial cavity, with the most common site being the fallopian tube (97%), followed by the ovary (3.2%) and the abdomen (1.3%) (9).

Ectopic pregnancy typically presents 6 to 8 weeks after the last normal menstrual period but can present earlier or later. Classical symptoms and signs of ectopic pregnancy are pain, vaginal bleeding and amenorrhoea. Haemodynamic instability and cervical motion tenderness may indicate rupture or imminent rupture of an ectopic pregnancy. If the woman is haemodynamically stable, transvaginal ultrasound is the initial test of choice.

If undiagnosed or untreated, it may lead to maternal death due to rupture of the implantation site and intraperitoneal haemorrhage (10).

Fifteen to 20% of all ectopic pregnancies occur in women with no known risk factors. However, a number of risk factors have been identified (9). Most risk factors are associated with prior damage to the fallopian tube (10). Documented tubal pathology includes previous surgery (21-fold increased risk) (11), pelvic infections (twofold to fourfold increased risk) and possibly endometriosis (12,13).

The role endometriosis plays as a risk factor for ectopic pregnancy is still heavily debated. Data presented from Aberdeen Royal Infirmary UK show that women with endometriosis have an increased risk of miscarriage, ectopic pregnancy and pregnancy complications (14). Some authors describe an increased incidence of ectopic pregnancy in women with endometriosis (12,13,15,16), with some suggesting the risk is doubled or tripled (14). Many authors do not include it as a strong or independent risk factor (17,18). It is believed that the presence of endometriosis may disrupt egg transportation (19) and this results in a complication, as the pregnancy advances, causing rupture of the fallopian tube resulting in major internal bleeding, which can be a life-threatening condition. Endometriosis-associated peritoneal inflammation complication also alters tubal physiology and causes a subsequent risk for ectopic pregnancy.

f. *Surgical complications*: Any type of surgery for endometriosis carries a risk of complications. Most of the time the complications are not serious and can include wound infection, bruising around the wound and bleeding.

The risk of complications depends on the type of surgery and severity of the condition.

Multiple procedures, surgery to remove adhesions and surgery to remove blockage from ureter carry increasing risk of complications.

The most serious complications can be a deep vein thrombosis (DVT), pulmonary embolism (PE), severe internal bleeding and damage to ureter, bladder, fallopian tube or bowel. Surgery for endometriosis that is around or inside the bladder can result in damage to the bladder, which can result in urostomy.

g. *Incomplete excision or ablation*: An incomplete excision or ablation can cause complications like bleeding, scar tissue or even infertility (20).

Prospective data indicates that recurrence rate after surgery ranges from 10–50% at 1 year and increases over time, resulting in more surgical interventions, increasing complications (3).

h. *Small bowel obstruction*: Endometriosis that affects the small bowel is rare, but a possible complication is a small bowel obstruction. It could be partial or total blockage of the small intestine. The scarring and inflammation of endometriosis cause bowel obstruction.

Small bowel obstruction can be a life-threatening complication without treatment, but prompt treatment can promote a good outcome.

i. *Chronic pain*: Chronic pain is one of the most common complications of endometriosis. In fact, 75% of people with endometriosis report experiencing pain. Many people with endometriosis experience painful menstrual periods and pain during or after sexual intercourse. The pain in some people with endometriosis is chronic (long-term), especially pain in their pelvis.

In some women, pain from endometriosis may become chronic even when visible disease has been removed (3).

The pain is linked to swelling and inflammation. The endometrial tissue often bleeds monthly, just as the endometrial tissue in your uterus does. However, since this blood can't flow out from the body, it causes pain and swelling. In addition, some of the surgical complications, including adhesions, can also cause pain.

j. *Mental health*: Having fertility issues, a serious complication of endometriosis, can result in a detrimental effect on mental health.

Living with the pain and discomfort of endometriosis can result in depression and anxiety. More than two-thirds of people with endometriosis report having psychological distress (21). Managing the symptoms of endometriosis may help with the mental health, but it's also important to refer the patient for specific mental health treatment.

k. *Reduced quality of life*: Symptomatic endometriosis can have a significant and sometimes severe impact on the woman's quality of life including work productivity, relationships, sexual health, fitness and daily living (22,23).

According to the World Health Organization (WHO), quality of life (QoL) is defined as a multidimensional construct of the individual perception of one's position in life in the context of culture and value systems about goals, expectations, standards and concerns (24). Painful symptoms and infertility, common complications of endometriosis, alone or combined, reduce QoL, impacting on all aspects of a woman's life such as daily activities, employment and work productivity, mood, social and sexual relationships and family planning (25). Several types of instruments are available to evaluate the multiple domains of QoL. A recent review (26) shows that the two scales most frequently used are the Short Form 36 Health Survey Questionnaire (SF-36) and Endometriosis Health Profile Questionaire (EHP-30) and that the most validated scales were SF-36 and EuroQual 5D (EQ-5D) for general questionnaires and EHP-30 and its abbreviated form EHP-5 for specific ones (26).

The SF-36 is used to indicate the health status of particular populations to help with service planning and to measure the impact of clinical and social interventions. NICE prefers to use utility values based on the EQ-5D questionnaire developed by EuroQol. The EQ-5D-5L is the latest version of the EQ-5D with five response options (e.g.,

"Regarding Pain/Discomfort—I have no pain or discomfort/I have slight pain or discomfort/I have moderate pain or discomfort/I have severe pain or discomfort").

Endometriosis-related symptoms can affect the sexual life of women with a decrease in the number and quality of coitus and compromising overall sexual activity, self-esteem and sexual satisfaction (27). The impairment of sex life is one of the main complications that compromises QoL of women with endometriosis, as shown in a market research survey conducted on 2,753 women with symptomatic or asymptomatic disease (28). The negative impact of endometriosis complications on sex life is mainly caused by dyspareunia, chronic pelvic pain and psychological factors, mostly depression (29,30).

PROGNOSIS DUE TO COMPLICATIONS

The prognosis of endometriosis is variable. For the majority of women, symptoms can be controlled with hormonal treatment (31); however, some women may have complex needs and require long-term support (32). Prospective data indicates that recurrence after surgery ranges from 10–50% at 1 year and increases over time (3). Observational studies in untreated women with infertility suggests that endometriotic deposits can regress spontaneously in up to 30% of women and progress is around 50% over 6–12 months (3). It is unclear whether endometriosis is always progressive, remains stable or improves with time (32).

An association between ovarian cancer and endometriosis has been suggested in some studies. The National Institute for Health and Care Excellence (NICE) undertook a systematic review to determine whether there is an increased risk of cancer of reproductive organs in women with endometriosis compared with those without endometriosis (32). The most consistent of the systematic review results were related to a possible small increased risk of ovarian cancer in women with endometriosis compared with women without endometriosis. But the evidence is limited, and the risk cannot be quantified in absolute terms as per NICE Guidelines and no recommendations are made in NICE Guidelines (32).

KEY POINT SUMMARY

- Fertility problems are among the major complications. Endometriosis is commonly associated with infertility, with a prevalence of 25–40% in infertile women compared with 0.5–5% in fertile women.

- Chronic pelvic pain due to adhesion formation may occur due to endometriosis or secondary to infection or complications of surgery. In some women, pain from endometriosis may become chronic even when visible disease is removed: a long-term complication.
- Complete or partial bowel obstruction can occur as a complication related to adhesion formation or circumferential endometriotic deposits.
- Symptomatic endometriosis with reduced quality of life is another long-term complication affecting mental health, relationships, sexuality and work productivity.

REFERENCES

1. El-Kader A, Gonied A, Mohamed M, et al. Impact of endometriosis-related adhesions on quality of life among infertile women. *Int J Fertil Steril* 2019;13(1):72–76.
2. Macer M, Taylor H. Endometriosis and infertility: A review of the pathogenesis and treatment of endometriosis-associated infertility. *Obstet Gynecol Clin North Am* 2012;39(4):535–49.
3. Hickey M, Ballard K, Farquhar C. Endometriosis. *BMJ* 2014;348:g1752.
4. Tanbo T, Fedorcsak P. Endometriosis-associated infertility: Aspects of pathophysiological mechanisms and treatment options. *Acta Obstet Gynecol Scand* 2017;96(6):659–67.
5. American Society for Reproductive Medicine Practice Committee. Endometriosis and infertility: A committee opinion. *Fertil Steril* 2012;98(3):591–98.
6. Johnson NP, Hummelshoj L. World Endometriosis Society Montpellier Consortium: Consensus on current management of endometriosis. *Hum Reprod* 2013;228:1552–68.
7. Wu L, Wu Q, Liu L. Oral contraceptive pills for endometriosis after conservative surgery: A systematic review and meta-analysis. *Gynecol Endocrinol* 2013;29:883–90.
8. Bayoglu Tekin Y, Dilbaz B, Altinbas SK, et al. Postoperative medical treatment of chronic pelvic pain related to severe endometriosis: Levonorgestrel-releasing intrauterine system versus gonadotropin-releasing hormone analogue. *Fertil Steril* 2011;95:492–6.
9. Shaw JL, Dey SK, Critchley HO, et al. Current knowledge of the aetiology of human tubal ectopic pregnancy. *Hum Reprod Update* 2010;16:432–44.
10. Doyle MB, DeCherney AH, Diamond MP. Epidemiology and etiology of ectopic pregnancy. *Obstet Gynecol Clin North Am* 1991;18:1–17.
11. Ankum WM, Mol BW, Van der Veen F, et al. Risk factors for ectopic pregnancy: A meta-analysis. *Fertil Steril* 1996;65(6):1093–9.
12. Coste J, Bouyer J, Job-Spira N. Construction of composite scales for risk assessment in epidemiology: An application to ectopic pregnancy. *Am J Epidemiol* 1977;145:278–89.
13. Job-Spira N, Collet P, Coste J, et al. Risk factors for ectopic pregnancy: Results of a case control study in the RhoneAlpes region. *Contracept Fertil Sex* 1993;21(4):307–12.
14. Kmietowicz Z. Endometriosis is linked to greater risk of complications in pregnancy and birth, study finds. *BMJ* 2015;350:h3252.

15. Tuomivaara L, Kauppila A. Ectopic pregnancy: A case control study of aetiological risk factors. *Arch Gynecol Obstet* 1988;243(1):5–11.
16. Bogdanskiene G, Berlingieri P, Grudzinskas JG. Association between ectopic pregnancy and pelvic endometriosis. *Int J Gynaecol Obstet* 2006;92:157–8.
17. Karande VC, Flood JT, Heard N, et al. Analysis of ectopic pregnancies resulting from in-vitro fertilization and embryo transfer. *Hum Reprod* 1991;6(3):446–9.
18. Cohen J, Mayaux MJ, Guihard-Moscato ML, et al. In-vitro fertilization and embryo transfer: A collaborative study of 1163 pregnancies on the incidence and risk factors of ectopic pregnancies. *Hum Reprod* 1986;1(4):255–8.
19. Stoppler M. *Ectopic pregnancy.* www.medicinenet.com/ectopic_pregnancy/page2.htm (accessed 10 Jan 2024).
20. Cao Q, Lu F, Feng WW, et al. Comparison of complete and incomplete excision of deep infiltrating endometriosis. *Int J Clin Exp Med* 2015;8(11):21497–506.
21. American Psychiatric Association. How endometriosis, a common, painful condition many women face, can impact mental health.
22. All Party Parliamentary Group on Endometriosis, Endometriosis UK. *Endometriosis in the UK: Time for change.* London: Endometriosis UK, 2020. www.endometriosis-uk.org/sites/default/files/files/Endometriosis%20APPG%20Report%20Oct%202020.pdf (accessed 2 Jan 2024).
23. Endometriosis: What are the complications and prognosis? Last revised in Oct 2023 Hickey et al, 2014; NICE, 2017.
24. Carr A, Higginson I, Robinson PG. Quality of Life. *BMJ* 2003;vii. London, UK. 133p [Google Scholar]
25. Moradi M., Parker M., Sneddon A., et al. Impact of endometriosis on women's lives: A qualitative study. *BMC Womens Health* 2014;14:123. doi:10.1186/1472-6874-14-123. [PMC free article] [PubMed] [CrossRef] [Google Scholar]
26. Bourdel N, Chauvet P, Billone V, et al. Systematic review of quality of life measures in patients with endometriosis. *PLoS One* 2019;14:e0208464. doi:10.1371/journal.pone.0208464. [PMC free article] [PubMed] [CrossRef] [Google Scholar]
27. Mabrouk M, Del Forno S, Spezzano A, et al. Painful love: Superficial dyspareunia and three dimensional transperineal ultrasound evaluation of pelvic floor muscle in women with endometriosis. *J Sex Marital Ther* 2019:1–10. doi:10.1080/0092623X.2019.1676852. [PubMed] [CrossRef] [Google Scholar]
28. Bernuit D, Ebert AD, Halis G, et al. Female perspectives on endometriosis: Findings from the uterine bleeding and pain women's research study. *J Endometr* 2011;3:73–85. doi:10.5301/JE.2011.8525. [CrossRef] [Google Scholar]
29. La Rosa VL, De Franciscis P, Barra F, et al. Sexuality in women with endometriosis: A critical narrative review. *Minerva Med* 2019. doi:10.23736/S0026-4806.19.06299-2. [PubMed] [CrossRef] [Google Scholar]
30. La Rosa VL, Barra F, Chiofalo B, et al. An overview on the relationship between endometriosis and infertility: The impact on sexuality and psychological wellbeing. *J Psychosom Obstet Gynaecol* 2019:1–5. doi:10.1080/0167482X.2019.1659775. [PubMed] [CrossRef] [Google Scholar]
31. Coleman L, Overton C. GPs have key role in early diagnosis of endometriosis. *Practitioner* 2015;259(1780):13. [Abstract]
32. NICE. *Endometriosis: Diagnosis and management.* National Institute for Health and Care Excellence. 2017. www.nice.org.uk

FURTHER READING

All Party Parliamentary Group on Endometriosis, Endometriosis UK. *Endometriosis in the UK: Time for change*. London: Endometriosis UK, 2020. www.endometriosis-uk.org/sites/default/files/files/Endometriosis%20APPG%20Report%20Oct%202020.pdf (accessed 12 Jan 2023)

BMJ. *Endometriosis*. BMJ Best Practice. 2019. www.bestpractice.bmj.com

Endometriosis-complications-NHS. www.nhs.uk/conditions/endometriosis

Hickey M, Ballard K, Farquhar C. Endometriosis. *BMJ* 2014;348:g1752

NICE. *Endometriosis: Diagnosis and management*. National Institute for Health and Care Excellence. 2017. www.nice.org.uk [Free Full-text]

NICE. *Endometriosis (Quality standard)*. National Institute for Health and Care Excellence. 2018b. www.nice.org.uk [Free Full-text]

CHAPTER 15

Endometriosis-Associated Infertility

....

Although endometriosis does not necessarily cause infertility, it can reduce fertility in many women. This does not mean that women with endometriosis cannot get pregnant; it means they may have a more challenging time getting pregnant.

Endometriosis is a progressive condition, which means it can gradually worsen over time. As more and more patches of endometriosis tissue grow in the pelvis and abdominal areas, they can block the reproductive organs, which can make it harder for the sperm to reach the egg.

It is important to remember that having endometriosis does not automatically mean that she will never be able to have children. Rather, it means that she may have more problems in getting pregnant. Endometriosis does not equal infertility!

Many women with endometriosis have children without difficulty, and many others become pregnant eventually—though it may take time and may require the help of surgery or assisted reproductive technologies or both.

Many theories have been proposed to explain why it is harder for women with endometriosis to conceive. However, none have been proven. It is possible that there are several causes and that different causes are relevant in different women. Some of the causes include:

- Pelvic adhesions inhibiting the movement of the egg down the fallopian tube

DOI: 10.1201/9781032684819-21

- Poor quality eggs
- Chemicals produced by the endometriosis inhibit the movement of the ovum down the fallopian tube
- Inflammation in the pelvis caused by endometriosis stimulates the production of cells that attack the sperm and shorten their life span
- Anovulation, which may also occur in women without endometriosis (1)

Miscarriage: There is no evidence that endometriosis causes women to have repeated miscarriages (2). Also, there is no evidence that treating endometriosis results in women having fewer miscarriages (3,4).

TYPES OF ENDOMETRIOSES AFFECTING FERTILITY

- *Superficial peritoneal*: Superficial peritoneal lesions are classified as stage I or II endometriosis. Despite superficial peritoneal lesion being the least severe form of endometriosis, some women may find conceiving difficult.

- *Endometriomas*: These are cysts that grow on the surface of or inside the ovaries. These are dark, fluid-filled sacs called chocolate cysts.

  When a person has endometrioma, they usually have stage III or stage IV of endometriosis. This means they may begin developing scar tissue on the fallopian tubes and ovaries. Endometriomas can greatly impact fertility due to their damaging effect on ovarian tissue, which may lead to issues with ovulation.

- *Deep-infiltrating endometriosis*: This is the most severe form of endometriosis, classified as stage IV. In deep-infiltrating endometriosis, endometrial-like tissue grows on organs near the uterus, such as the vagina, bladder and bowel. In addition to endometriomas, woman with stage IV endometriosis may have extensive scarring in the ovaries, uterus and rectum.

If a person has already undergone previous cyst removal surgeries, that can have an additional impact on getting pregnant as they may have also lost a significant number of eggs.

It is important to note that while a person may no longer be able to conceive naturally at this stage, they may become pregnant with IVF treatment.

THE ENDOMETRIOSIS FERTILITY INDEX (EFI)

The Endometriosis Fertility Index (EFI) is a 10-point scale, developed in 2010 (see Figure 15.1) (5), that can tell how likely a woman is to get pregnant without medical intervention.

The score can predict their likelihood of getting pregnant, and it can help individuals and doctors to make the best decisions for their fertility.

In the EFI, 5 out of 10 points are based on patient characteristics such as age, duration of infertility and prior pregnancy. Parts of the revised American Society of Reproductive Medicine (rASRM) staging (endometriosis lesion score (< or ≥16) and total rASRM score (< or ≥71)) account for 2 out of 10 points, and the remaining 3 points are based on the end-of-surgery qualitative visual assessment by the surgeon of the adnexal function ("least function score"). Currently, the EFI is a thoroughly validated scoring system predicting pregnancy rates without using assisted reproduction technique (ART) treatment in postoperative endometriosis patients who suffer from infertility, taking into account all endometriosis rASRM stages (5–7), although its predictive performance remains modest (6).

The EFI is considered a valid tool to make clinical decisions on postoperative fertility management (6,8). Consequently, the EFI has been adopted by the World Endometriosis Society (WES) in their consensus on the classification of endometriosis (9). Of note, the surgical adnexal "least function score" (max. 3 points) is the most important contributor to the EFI score, without evidence that the information not captured in the EFI least function score is redundant (6). The EFI score ranges from 0–10, with 0 representing the poorest prognosis and 10 the best prognosis. Half of the points come from the historical factors and half from the surgical factors. Uterine abnormality was not included in the score.

EFI is a simple, robust and validated clinical tool that predicts pregnancy rate (PR) for patients after surgical staging of endometriosis. The EFI is very useful in developing treatment plans in infertile patients with endometriosis. Its use provides reassurance to those patients with good prognoses and avoids wasted time and treatment for those with poor prognoses.

ENDOMETRIOSIS FERTILITY INDEX (EFI)
SURGERY FORM

LEAST FUNCTION (LF) SCORE AT CONCLUSION OF SURGERY

Score	Description		Left	Right
4 =	Normal	Fallopian Tube	☐	☐
3 =	Mild Dysfunction			
2 =	Moderate Dysfunction	Fimbria	☐	☐
1 =	Severe Dysfunction			
0 =	Absent or Nonfunctional	Ovary	☐	☐

To calculate the LF score, add together the lowest score for the left side and the lowest score for the right side. If an ovary is absent on one side, the LF score is obtained by doubling the lowest score on the side with the ovary.

Lowest Score	☐	+	☐	=	☐
	Left		Right		LF Score

ENDOMETRIOSIS FERTILITY INDEX (EFI)

Historical Factors			Surgical Factors		
Factor	Description	Points	Factor	Description	Points
Age			LF Score		
	If age is < 35 years	2		If LF Score = 7 to 8 (high score)	3
	If age is 36 to 39 years	1		If LF Score = 4 to 6 (moderate score)	2
	If age is > 40 years	0		If LF Score = 1 to 3 (low score)	0
Years Infertile			AFS Endometriosis Score		
	If years infertile is < 3	2		If AFS Endometriosis Lesion Score is < 16	1
	If years infertile is > 3	0		If AFS Endometriosis Lesion Score is > 16	0
Prior Pregnancy			AFS Total Score		
	If there is a history of a prior pregnancy	1		If AFS total score is < 71	1
	If there is no history of prior pregnancy	0		If AFS total score is > 71	0
Total Historical Factors			**Total Surgical Factors**		

EFI = TOTAL HISTORICAL FACTORS + TOTAL SURGICAL FACTORS:	☐	+	☐	=	☐
		Historical		Surgical	EFI Score

ESTIMATED PERCENT PREGNANT BY EFI SCORE

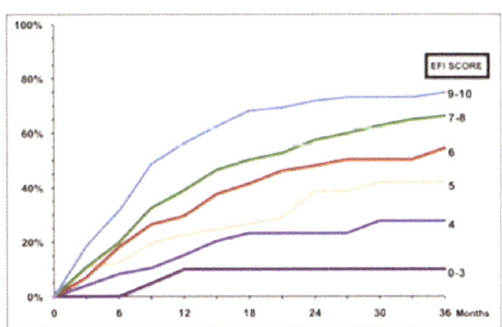

FIGURE 15.1 Endometriosis Fertility Index (EFI) surgery form. (Reprinted from *Fertility and Sterility,* Vol 94, Adamson G.D. and Pasta D.J., Endometriosis Fertility Index: the new, validated endometriosis staging system, 1609–1615, 2010, with permission from Elsevier.)

FERTILITY TREATMENT OPTIONS

Hormonal Treatment

Minimal–Mild Endometriosis

In women with minimal–mild endometriosis, hormonal drugs are not an effective treatment for endometriosis-related infertility. Therefore, they should not be used to improve fertility in women with minimal to mild endometriosis (10).

Moderate–Severe Endometriosis

In women with more severe disease, no published studies have looked at the effect of hormonal treatment on infertility. However, it is assumed that they are not effective, so they should not be used to improve infertility in women with moderate–severe disease (11).

No evidence exists of the benefit of suppression of ovarian function in women with endometriosis-associated infertility who wish to conceive (12). Following surgery for endometriosis, women seeking pregnancy should not be treated with postoperative hormone suppression with the sole purpose of enhancing future pregnancy rates.

Surgical Treatment Options to Increase the Chance of Natural Pregnancy

Aim

Surgery for endometriosis-related infertility aims to remove any endometriosis and adhesions present.

If the endometriosis has damaged any organs or resulted in them being stuck down in abnormal positions, the surgery will also try to repair the damage and restore the anatomy of the organs to as close as possible to their normal positioning (13).

Several treatment options are available for people with endometriosis who have not become pregnant after 6–12 months of trying.

The treatment depends on the stage and type of endometriosis a person has.

Minimal–Mild Endometriosis

In women with minimal–mild endometriosis, laparoscopic surgery is an effective treatment for endometriosis-related infertility, as it leads to better pregnancy rates than a diagnostic laparoscopy alone.

Moderate quality evidence from a Cochrane meta-analysis of three RCTs in a total of 528 participants shows that laparoscopic treatment (ablation or excision) of superficial peritoneal endometriosis increases viable intrauterine pregnancy rates compared with diagnostic laparoscopy only (odds ratio 1.89, 95% confidence interval 1.25 to 2.86) (14).

Moderate–Severe Endometriosis

In women with moderate–severe endometriosis, no well-designed studies have looked at the effect of surgery on pregnancy rates (13).

However, three studies seem to suggest that the more severe the endometriosis, the lower the pregnancy rates following surgery (3,15,16). In other words, it seems that women with severe endometriosis are less likely to become pregnant following surgery than women with mild or moderate endometriosis.

Nevertheless, some gynaecologists believe that women with the most severe forms of endometriosis have the greatest improvements in pregnancy rates following surgery (17). In other words, surgery seems to increase their chances of becoming pregnant proportionally more than women with less severe endometriosis.

In the later stages of endometriosis, IVF is likely to be recommended.

Ovarian Endometriomas

There is considerable debate about how large ovarian endometriomas in women with endometriosis-related infertility should be treated (9). The three main treatments are:

- Draining the endometrioma
- Draining and coagulating (burning the lining of) the endometrioma
- Excising (remove by cutting out) the endometrioma from the ovary

Several studies indicate that laparoscopically excising large endometriomas greater than 4 cm in diameter leads to increased pregnancy rates and decreased recurrence rates compared with draining and coagulating the endometrioma (18–21).

CHOOSING THE APPROPRIATE TREATMENT OPTION

No data was found on live birth rates, and the effect on ectopic pregnancy and miscarriage rates is unclear. No published RCTs have assessed fertility outcomes after surgery for ovarian or deep disease, and surgery is generally recommended only in the presence of painful symptoms (22).

Use of the Endometriosis Fertility Index to support decision-making for the most appropriate option to achieve pregnancy after surgery (for example, women who may benefit from medically assisted reproduction) has been recently suggested (23).

Medically Assisted Reproduction

There is low-quality evidence that viable intrauterine pregnancy rates are increased in women with superficial peritoneal endometriosis if they undergo intrauterine insemination with ovarian stimulation, instead of expectant management or intrauterine insemination alone.

In one RCT of 103 participants randomized either to ovarian stimulation with gonadotrophins and intrauterine insemination treatment or to expectant management, the live birth rate was 5.6 (95% confidence interval 1.18 to 17.4) times higher in the treated couples (24).

In women with ovarian or deep endometriosis, the benefit of ovarian stimulation with intrauterine insemination is unclear. No RCTs have evaluated the efficacy of assisted reproductive technology (ART) versus no intervention in women with endometriosis.

Doing surgery before ART for infertility associated with superficial peritoneal endometriosis is not recommended, as the evidence suggesting benefit is based on a single retrospective study of low quality (25) (and is not supported by indirect evidence from multiple studies comparing outcomes in women with surgically treated endometriosis and those managed without surgery) (26).

Doing surgery for ovarian endometrioma before ART to improve live birth rates is also not recommended. Current evidence shows no benefit, and surgery is likely to have a negative effect on ovarian reserve (27,28).

In addition, no evidence shows that doing surgical excision of deep endometriosis before ART improves reproductive outcomes, and this should be reserved for women with concomitant painful symptoms.

In Vitro Fertilization

Currently, IVF is the most successful treatment for infertile women with endometriosis and includes a few steps.

The first step is ovarian stimulation initiated by drugs and the suppression of the menstrual cycle using other medications. After follicle stimulation, monitoring is performed at certain intervals to evaluate the follicle's growth. Once the follicles have reached a proper dimension, medication is administered to induce the final stage of maturation of the oocyte.

The next step implies collecting the egg, followed by the fertilization process. The fertilized egg is cultured in a specific media for a few days and then the embryos are transferred into the uterus (29).

A meta-analysis has shown that patients suffering from endometrioma who underwent IVF had comparable live birth rates as well as clinical pregnancy and miscarriage rates when compared to women who were not affected by this disease, even though the mean number of oocytes and the antral follicle count were lower, and the risk of cycle cancellation was increased in women with endometrioma (30).

Studies reported that there is no difference regarding IVF results between patients with reduced ovarian reserve after ovarian surgery and those with reduced ovarian reserve without prior endometrioma surgical treatment (31).

Systemic review reported that second-line conservative surgery for recurrent endometriosis has a negative effect on the IVF outcomes. The number of mature oocytes retrieved following IVF procedure and high-quality embryos was considerably reduced after second-line conservative surgery than after the initial conservative surgical intervention.

Second-line surgery seems to significantly diminish the ovarian reserve; therefore, this procedure should be attentively considered as an alternative therapeutic method of women who desire a future pregnancy (32,33).

Support for Endometriosis and Infertility

Endometriosis is a painful, progressive condition that can be difficult to cope with. People struggling to get pregnant with the condition may feel isolated and discouraged, especially if they have been trying for a number of years without success. Living with endometriosis can be difficult, and support groups and resources can help those who are struggling.

KEY POINT SUMMARY

- For those with superficial endometriosis (where tissue attaches to the peritoneum), there is evidence that laparoscopic surgery leads to better pregnancy rates, and it can improve the chances of becoming pregnant naturally if you have had problems conceiving.

- For those with deep endometriosis (where the bowel, bladder or ureter is involved), there has been little research on the effect of surgery on pregnancy rates.
- In general, pain improves during pregnancy but may return after giving birth as periods return. There are reports of individuals who had more pain in the first few months of pregnancy.
- Pregnancy does not cure endometriosis.
- Miscarriage is a common problem in all pregnancies, regardless of endometriosis. Miscarriage occurs in around 1 in 5 pregnancies, and if one has endometriosis, the risk increases to around 1 in 4.
- Ectopic pregnancies are less common than miscarriages, with around 1 in 80 to 100 pregnancies ending up as ectopic. But research has shown that in those with endometriosis, the risk is more than doubled.

REFERENCES

1. Kennedy S. *The patient's essential guide to endometriosis.* United Kingdom: Alden, 2003: p. 42.
2. Vercammen EE, D'Hooghe TM. Endometriosis and recurrent pregnancy loss. *Semin Reprod Med* 2000;18:363–8.
3. Marcoux S, Maheux R, Berube S. Laparoscopic surgery in infertile women with minimal or mild endometriosis: Canadian Collaborative Group on Endometriosis. *N Engl J Med* 1997;337:217–22.
4. Parazzini F. Ablation of lesions or no treatment in minimal-mild endometriosis in infertile women: A randomized trial: Gruppo Italiano per lo Studio dell'Endometriosi. *Hum Reprod* 1999;14:1332–4.
5. Adamson GD, Pasta DJ. Endometriosis fertility index: The new, validated endometriosis staging system. *Fertil Steril* 2010;94:1609–15.
6. Tomassetti C, Geysenbergh B, Meuleman C, et al. External validation of the endometriosis fertility index (EFI) staging system for predicting non-ART pregnancy after endometriosis surgery *Human Reprod* 2013;28:1280–8.
7. Vesali S, Razavi M, Rezaeinejad M, et al. Endometriosis fertility index for predicting non-assisted reproductive technology pregnancy after endometriosis surgery: A systematic review and meta-analysis. *BJOG* 2020;127:800–9.
8. Adamson GD. Endometriosis fertility index: Is it better than the present staging systems? *Curr Opin Obstet Gynecol* 2013;25:186–92.
9. Johnson NP, Hummelshoj L, Adamson GD, et al. World Endometriosis Society consensus on the classification of endometriosis. *Hum Reprod* 2017;32:315–24.
10. Hughes E, Fedorkow D, Collins J, et al. Ovulation suppression for endometriosis (Cochrane Review). *Cochrane Database Syst Rev* 2007;3. doi:10.1002/14651858.CD000155.pub2 Art. No.: CD000155.
11. *ESHRE Guidelines.* 2007. http://guidelines.endometriosis.org
12. Hughes E, Brown J, Collins JJ, et al. Ovulation suppression for endometriosis. *Cochrane Database Syst Rev* 2007;2007(3):CD000155. pmid:17636607
13. Speroff L, Fritz M. *Clinical gynecologic endocrinology and infertility.* United States of America: Lippincott Williams & Wilkins, 2005: p. 1014.

14. Bafort C, Beebeejaun Y, Tomassetti C, et al. Laparoscopic surgery for endometriosis. *Cochrane Database Syst Rev* 2020;10:CD011031. pmid:33095458
15. Kennedy S. *The patient's essential guide to endometriosis.* United Kingdom: Alden, 2003: p. 42.
16. Vercammen EE, D'Hooghe TM. Endometriosis and recurrent pregnancy loss. *Semin Reprod Med* 2000;18:363–8.
17. Parazzini F. Ablation of lesions or no treatment in minimal-mild endometriosis in infertile women: A randomized trial: Gruppo Italiano per lo Studio dell'Endometriosi. *Hum Reprod* 1999;14:1332–4.
18. Hughes E, Fedorkow D, Collins J, et al. Ovulation suppression for endometriosis (Cochrane Review). *Cochrane Database Syst Rev* 2007;3. doi:10.1002/14651858.CD000155.pub2 Art. No.: CD000155.
19. *ESHRE Guidelines.* 2007. http://guidelines.endometriosis.org
20. Jacobson TZ, Barlow DH, Koninckx PR, et al. Laparoscopic surgery for subfertility associated with endometriosis (Cochrane Review). *Cochrane Database Syst Rev* 2002;4. doi:10.1002/14651858.CD001398 Art. No.: CD001398.
21. Adamson GD, Hurd SJ, Pasta DJ, et al. Laparoscopic endometriosis treatment: Is it better? *Fertil Steril* 1993;59:35–44.
22. Becker CM, Bokor A, Heikinheimo O, et al. ESHRE Endometriosis Guideline Group. ESHRE guideline: Endometriosis. *Hum Reprod Open* 2022;2022:hoac009. doi:10.1093/hropen/hoac009 pmid:35350465 [CrossRef] [PubMed] [Google Scholar]
23. Bafort C, Beebeejaun Y, Tomassetti C, et al. Laparoscopic surgery for endometriosis. *Cochrane Database Syst Rev* 2020;10:CD011031. pmid:33095458 [PubMed] [Google Scholar]
24. Tummon IS, Asher LJ, Martin JS, et al. Randomized controlled trial of superovulation and insemination for infertility associated with minimal or mild endometriosis. *Fertil Steril* 1997;68:8–12. doi:10.1016/S0015-0282(97)81467-7 pmid:9207576 [CrossRef] [PubMed] [Web of Science] [Google Scholar]
25. Opøien HK, Fedorcsak P, Byholm T, et al. Complete surgical removal of minimal and mild endometriosis improves outcome of subsequent IVF/ICSI treatment. *Reprod Biomed Online* 2011;23:389–95. doi:10.1016/j.rbmo.2011.06.002 pmid:21764382 [CrossRef] [PubMed] [Web of Science] [Google Scholar]
26. Hamdan M, Omar SZ, Dunselman G, et al. Influence of endometriosis on assisted reproductive technology outcomes: A systematic review and meta-analysis. *Obstet Gynecol* 2015;125:79–88. doi:10.1097/AOG.0000000000000592 pmid:25560108 [CrossRef] [PubMed] [Google Scholar]
27. Hamdan M, Dunselman G, Li TC, et al. The impact of endometrioma on IVF/ICSI outcomes: A systematic review and meta-analysis. *Hum Reprod Update* 2015;21:809–25. doi:10.1093/humupd/dmv035 pmid:26168799 [CrossRef] [PubMed] [Google Scholar]
28. Nickkho-Amiry M, Savant R, Majumder K, et al. The effect of surgical management of endometrioma on the IVF/ICSI outcomes when compared with no treatment? A systematic review and meta-analysis. *Arch Gynecol Obstet* 2018;297:1043–57. doi:10.1007/s00404-017-4640-1 pmid:29344847 [CrossRef] [PubMed] [Google Scholar]
29. Farquhar C, Rishworth JR, Brown J, et al. Assisted reproductive technology: An overview of Cochrane Reviews. *Cochrane Database Syst Rev* 2015. [CrossRef] [PubMed]
30. Hamdan M, Dunselman G, Li TC, et al. The impact of endometrioma on IVF/ICSI outcomes: A systematic review and meta-analysis. *Hum Reprod Update* 2015;21:809–25.

31. Gallinelli A, Chiossi G, Giannella L, et al. Different concentrations of inter-leukins in the peritoneal fluid of women with endometriosis: Relationships with lymphocyte subsets. *Gynecol Endocrinol* 2004;18:144–51.
32. Vercellini P, Somigliana E, Viganò P, et al. The effect of second-line surgery on reproductive performance of women with recurrent endometriosis A sys-tematic review. *Acta Obstet Gynecol Scand* 2009;88:1074–82. [CrossRef] [PubMed]
33. Park H, Kim CH, Kim EY, et al. Effect of second-line surgery on in vitro fertilization outcome in infertile women with ovarian endometrioma recur-rence after primary conservative surgery for moderate to severe endometrio-sis. *Obstet Gynecol Sci* 2015;58:481–86.

FURTHER READING

Endometriosis: The experts' guide to treat, manage, and live well with your symp-toms by Professor Andrew Horne and Carol Pearson.
Fertility Network UK. https://fertilitynetworkuk.org/
Human Fertilisation and Embryology Authority (HFEA). www.hfea.gov.uk/
NICE. *Guideline* [NG73]: Endometriosis diagnosis and management. 2017. https://www.nice.org.uk/guidance/ng73
Royal College of Obstetricians and Gynaecologists (RCOG). www.rcog.org.uk/en/patients/fertility/

CHAPTER 16

Comorbidities in Women with Endometriosis

···

Endometriosis is a multisystem condition perhaps because of common pathogenesis or because of the chronic endogenous response to the presence of endometriotic lesions (1).

Women with endometriosis demonstrate a high incidence of gynaecological and non-gynaecological comorbidities and chronic conditions, which can be challenging for health professionals.

GYNAECOLOGICAL COMORBIDITIES

Women with endometriosis have a greater risk of presenting with gynaecological diseases, including uterine fibroids and adenomyosis (2,3).

Uterine fibroids (leiomyomata) are a common oestrogen-responsive gynaecological condition responsible for overlapping symptoms including subfertility and pelvic pain.

The coexisting gynaecologic conditions such as adenomyosis and uterine fibroids (2), as well as associations with endometrial cancer (4), can be influenced by diagnostic biases and failure to distinguish between diagnoses in women undergoing hysterectomy and those with an intact uterus (3,5).

Women with endometriosis are also at a greater risk of early natural menopause (6).

Varied degrees of comorbidity between endometriosis and fibroids ranging from 12 to 87.1% have been reported in retrospective studies (7). Despite the two pathologies having distinct developmental trajectories, the studies emphasize common genetic underpinnings that recent

DOI: 10.1201/9781032684819-22

genome-wide association studies (GWAS) meta-analyses have revealed that increase risk for both endometriosis and fibroids; on chromosome 1 encoding for CDC42 and WNT4, chromosome 2 for GREB1, chromosome 6 for SYNE1 and ESR1 and chromosome 11 for FSHB.

Given the substantial comorbidity between the conditions, it might be beneficial to factor in surgery for one condition when addressing the other, to avoid the need for repeating surgical procedures (7).

Ovarian Cancer

Endometriosis appears to be associated with some epithelial ovarian cancers (EOC) (8). Whether women with endometriosis are at risk for other types of cancers is unclear, but the overall risk appears to be low (9,10).

In a meta-analysis of 13 case-control studies including nearly 8,000 women with epithelial ovarian cancer, women with a self-reported history of endometriosis had three times the risk of clear cell epithelial ovarian cancer and double the risk of endometroid and low-grade serous epithelial ovarian cancer but no change in the risk of high grade serous or mucinous epithelial ovarian cancer (11).

Activation of oncogenic KRAS and P13K pathways and inactivation of tumor suppressor genes PTEN and ARID1A have been suggested as mechanisms for the transformation of endometriosis, particularly ovarian endometriomas, to malignancy (8). The risk of malignant transformation of endometriosis has been estimated at 1% of premenopausal women (12) and 1–2.5% for postmenopausal women (13,14).

In a study of women with postmenopausal endometriosis, 35% had different grades of metaplasia, hyperplasia and endometrioid carcinoma arising in ovarian endometriosis.

Endometriosis-associated epithelial ovarian cancers appear to develop in younger women and have a better prognosis than most cases of epithelial ovarian cancers. While there appears to be an association between endometriosis and epithelial ovarian cancers, endometriosis is not considered a premalignant lesion, and screening is not recommended. Also, there is no available data indicating that prophylactic removal of endometriosis lesions reduces the risk of epithelial ovarian cancers.

NON-GYNAECOLOGICAL COMORBIDITIES

Pelvic pain is the most common symptom of possible endometriosis, and women with endometriosis also have a high risk of co-occurring multi-site pain (15).

Local and systemic chronic inflammation can directly activate afferent nociceptive fibres and promote pelvic pain (16) although this does not explain the severity of painful symptoms that patients experience. Furthermore, endometriosis-induced chronic inflammation and immune dysregulation may also contribute to the endometriosis-associated subsequent risk of each of these comorbid conditions (17).

Comorbid Chronic Pain Conditions

Patients with endometriosis have a higher risk of presentation with comorbid chronic pain conditions such as:

- Fibromyalgia (18,19)
- Osteoarthritis (20)
- Psoriatic arthritis (21)
- Rheumatoid arthritis (20)
- Migraines (22,23)
- Bladder, bowel and back pain (24) (Nearly 50% of women with bladder pain syndrome or interstitial cystitis have endometriosis) (25,26)
- Dyschezia being potentially predictive of endometriosis (27)
- Irritable bowel syndrome (A common co-occurring diagnosis that reinforces the importance of awareness of endometriosis among gastroenterologists) (27,28)
- Greater risk of a subsequent diagnosis of malignancies, autoimmune diseases and cerebrovascular and cardiovascular conditions (4,6,20,29,30)

These conditions may share a common cause, or they may arise together owing to shared environmental or genetic factors. Also the occurrence of comorbid pain conditions could be due to changes in pain perception after repeated sensitization (31).

Risk of Melanoma

Among non-gynaecological cancers, melanoma skin cancer has been the most studied in relation to a history of endometriosis.

A diagnosis of endometriosis was associated with an increased risk of developing melanoma compared to those without endometriosis. It is important to acknowledge that the absolute increase in the risk of melanoma in women with endometriosis remains low, which should be considered when counselling women (32).

Significant positive correlation between melanoma and endometriosis with the identification of 27 genomic loci that are associated with the two diseases was found (33). The authors clearly state further and larger studies are needed to confirm or refute those findings (33).

Food Hypersensitivity and Endometriosis

It is suggested that there is a link between endometriosis and allergic hypersensitivities, including allergic and non-allergic food hypersensitivity.

No studies elucidated a statistically significant link between allergic food hypersensitivity alone and endometriosis. Therefore, based on a small number of studies with limited research quality, evidence does not support the existence of a link between endometriosis and allergic or non-allergic food hypersensitivity (34). Sufficiently powered evidence-based research is required, including information which better characterizes the patient's endometriosis symptoms, importantly the gastrointestinal sequalae, as well as specific allergic and non-allergic food hypersensitivities and method of diagnoses. Confirming a link between endometriosis and food hypersensitivities is an essential step forward in dispelling the many myths surrounding endometriosis and improving management of disease.

Asthma and Allergic Manifestations

The available evidence suggests that women with endometriosis may be more susceptible to allergic manifestations like eczema, hay fever, allergies to medication and allergy-related conditions such as asthma (35).

Psychiatric Comorbidities

Psychological factors have an important role in determining the severity of symptoms and the effectiveness of the treatments in patients with endometriosis.

Women with endometriosis are at risk for anxiety, depressive symptoms and other psychiatric disorders (36).

Since it is still unclear if these comorbidities are a result of endometriosis itself or other factors such as chronic pelvic pain, further studies are needed.

Most studies describe stress-related disorders, eating disorders, attention deficit hyperactivity disorders and personality disorders as being common among women with endometriosis, and some even suggest familial liability although the mechanistic causation requires to be investigated further as the generalizability of this data remains poor.

Overall, psychiatric comorbidities remain unreported and unsubstantiated except for a study (37) reporting reduced psychological functioning and quality of life (QoL) because of mental health difficulties, 56.4% of women with endometriosis fulfilled the clinical criteria for psychiatric disorders (37).

Atherosclerosis and Cardiovascular Disease

There is an increased oxidative stress and systemic chronic inflammation in the pathogenesis of both endometriosis and atherosclerosis. An elevated risk of atherosclerosis and coronary heart disease (CHD) has been hypothesized in women with endometriosis (38). This association has been strengthened by studies reporting a proatherogenic profile and increased subclinical atherosclerosis in women with endometriosis (39).

A study of over 116,000 women with stroke or heart disease reported that women with laparoscopically confirmed endometriosis had an increased risk of myocardial infarction (MI), coronary artery bypass graft (CABG), coronary angioplasty procedure/stent or combined CHD endpoints compared to women without endometriosis (40). The risk was also higher in women who underwent hysterectomy/oophorectomy compared to those who did not, which may explain some of the association between endometriosis and CHD.

However, more data are needed on the risk of CHD in women with endometriosis and benefits of CHD screening for these women.

Pregnancy

Endometriotic lesions and the symptoms often disappear or improve during pregnancy. However, decidualization of lesions does not make them biologically inactive.

Complications have been reported in pregnant women caused by endometriosis, including intestinal perforation (41), hemoperitoneum (42) acute appendicitis (43) and ruptured or infected ovarian endometrioma (44).

As these events are rare, no additional monitoring or interventions are recommended for pregnant women with a history of endometriosis.

Obstetric Outcomes

Endometriosis increases the risk of preterm birth (45). In a retrospective population-based study of over 82,000 pregnancies, endometriosis was associated with an increased risk of preterm birth, pre-eclampsia and cesarean section when compared with no endometriosis (45).

Increased risk of miscarriage, ectopic pregnancy, placenta previa, unexplained antepartum hemorrhage, postpartum hemorrhage and preterm birth has also been reported (46). Decreased or no change in the risk of hypertensive disorders of pregnancy in women with endometriosis has been reported (47).

The mechanism behind these associations is not known, and additional surveillance for pregnant women with known endometriosis is not advised (44).

KEY POINT SUMMARY

- The challenge for health professionals is increased further by growing observations indicating that people with endometriosis also demonstrate a high incidence of gynaecological and non-gynaecological comorbidities and chronic conditions.
- Irritable bowel syndrome is a common co-occurring diagnosis that reinforces the importance of awareness of endometriosis among gastroenterologists.
- Women with endometriosis have a greater risk of presenting with uterine fibroids and adenomyosis.
- They are also at greater risk of early natural menopause and cerebrovascular, cardiovascular and autoimmune diseases.
- Endometriosis-associated epithelial ovarian cancer appears to develop in younger women and has a better prognosis than most epithelial ovarian cancers.
- Endometriosis appears to negatively impact pregnancy outcome, particularly increasing the risk of preterm birth, miscarriages, ectopic pregnancy, unexplained antepartum and postpartum haemorrhage, preeclampsia and caesarean section delivery when compared with no endometriosis.

REFERENCES

1. Missmer SA. Commentary: Endometriosis—epidemiologic considerations for a potentially 'high-risk' population. *Int J Epidemiol* 2009;38:1154–5. doi:10.1093/ije/dyp249 pmid:19617382 [CrossRef] [PubMed] [Web of Science] [Google Scholar]
2. Gallagher CS, Mäkinen N, Harris HR, et al. Genome-wide association and epidemiological analyses reveal common genetic origins between uterine leiomyomata and endometriosis. *Nat Commun* 2019;10:4857. doi:10.1038/s41467-019-12536-4 pmid:31649266 [CrossRef] [PubMed] [Google Scholar]

3. Upson K, Missmer SA. Epidemiology of adenomyosis. *Semin Reprod Med* 2020;38:89–107. doi:10.1055/s-0040-1718920 pmid:33105509 [CrossRef] [PubMed] [Google Scholar]

4. Kvaskoff M, Mahamat-Saleh Y, Farland LV, et al. Endometriosis and cancer: A systematic review and meta-analysis. *Hum Reprod Update* 2021;27:393–420. doi:10.1093/humupd/dmaa045 pmid:33202017 [CrossRef] [PubMed] [Google Scholar]

5. Shafrir AL, Farland LV, Shah DK, et al. Risk for and consequences of endometriosis: A critical epidemiologic review. *Best Pract Res Clin Obstet Gynaecol* 2018;51:1–15. doi:10.1016/j.bpobgyn.2018.06.001 pmid:30017581 [CrossRef] [PubMed] [Google Scholar]

6. Thombre Kulkarni M, Shafrir A, Farland LV, et al. Association between laparoscopically confirmed endometriosis and risk of early natural menopause. *JAMA Netw Open* 2022;5:e2144391. doi:10.1001/jamanetworkopen.2021.44391 pmid:35061039 [CrossRef] [PubMed] [Google Scholar]

7. Uimari O, Nazri H, Tapmeier T. Endometriosis and uterine fibroids (leiomyomata): Comorbidity, risks and implications. *Front Reprod Health* 2021;3. doi:10.3389/frph.2021.750018 View all 6 Articles

8. Grandi G, Toss A, Cortesi L, et al. The association between endometriomas and ovarian cancer: Preventive effect of inhibiting ovulation and menstruation during reproductive life. *Biomed Res Int* 2015;2015:751571.

9. Somigliana E, Vigano' P, Parazzini F, et al. Association between endometriosis and cancer: A comprehensive review and a critical analysis of clinical and epidemiological evidence. *Gynecol Oncol* 2006;101:331.

10. Melin A, Sparen P, Berggvist A. The risk of cancer and the role of parity among women with endometriosis. *Hum Reprod* 2007;22:3021.

11. Pearce CL, Templeman C, Rossing MA, et al. Association between endometriosis and risk of histological subtypes of ovarian cancer: A pooled analysis of case-control studies. *Lancet Oncol* 2012;13:385.

12. Oxholm D, Knudsen UB, Kryger-Baggesen N, et al. Postmenopausal endometriosis. *Acta Obstet Gynecol Scand* 2007;86:1158.

13. Van Gorp T, Amant F, Neven P, et al. Endometriosis and the development of malignant tumours of the pelvis. A review of literature. *Best Pract Res Clin Obstet Gynaecol* 2004;18:349.

14. Sampson JA. Endometrial carcinoma of the ovary arising in endometrial tissue in that organ. *Arch Surg* 1925;10:1.

15. Yong PJ, Williams C, Bedaiwy MA, et al. A proposed platform for phenotyping endometriosis-associated pain: Unifying peripheral and central pain mechanisms. *Curr Obstet Gynecol Rep* 2020;9:89–97. doi:10.1007/s13669-020-00288-8. [CrossRef] [Google Scholar]

16. Morotti M, Vincent K, Brawn J, et al. Peripheral changes in endometriosis-associated pain. *Hum Reprod Update* 2014;20:717–36. doi:10.1093/humupd/dmu021 pmid:24859987 [CrossRef] [PubMed] [Google Scholar]

17. Zondervan KT, Becker CM, Koga K, et al. Endometriosis. *Nat Rev Dis Primers* 2018;4:9. doi:10.1038/s41572-018-0008-5 pmid:30026507 [CrossRef] [PubMed] [Google Scholar]

18. Coloma JL, Martínez-Zamora MA, Collado A, et al. Prevalence of fibromyalgia among women with deep infiltrating endometriosis. *Int J Gynaecol Obstet* 2019;146:157–63. doi:10.1002/ijgo.12822 pmid:30973964 [CrossRef] [PubMed] [Google Scholar]

19. Larrosa Pardo F, Bondesson E, Schelin MEC, et al. A diagnosis of rheumatoid arthritis, endometriosis or IBD is associated with later onset of fibromyalgia and chronic widespread pain. *Eur J Pain* 2019;23:1563–73.

doi:10.1002/ejp.1432 pmid:31131959 [CrossRef] [PubMed] [Google Scholar]

20. Shigesi N, Kvaskoff M, Kirtley S, et al. The association between endometriosis and autoimmune diseases: A systematic review and meta-analysis. *Hum Reprod Update* 2019;25:486–503. doi:10.1093/humupd/dmz014 pmid:31260048 [CrossRef] [PubMed] [Google Scholar]
21. Harris HR, Korkes KMN, Li T, et al. Endometriosis, psoriasis, and psoriatic arthritis: A prospective cohort study. *Am J Epidemiol* 2022;191:1050–60. doi:10.1093/aje/kwac009 pmid:35029650 [CrossRef] [PubMed] [Google Scholar]
22. Jenabi E, Khazaei S. Endometriosis and migraine headache risk: A meta-analysis. *Women Health* 2020;60:939–45. doi:10.1080/03630242.2020.1779905 pmid:32552576 [CrossRef] [PubMed] [Google Scholar]
23. Miller JA, Missmer SA, Vitonis AF, et al. Prevalence of migraines in adolescents with endometriosis. *Fertil Steril* 2018;109:685–90. doi:10.1016/j.fertnstert.2017.12.016 pmid:29605402 [CrossRef] [PubMed] [Google Scholar]
24. DiVasta AD, Vitonis AF, Laufer MR, et al. Spectrum of symptoms in women diagnosed with endometriosis during adolescence vs adulthood. *Am J Obstet Gynecol* 2018;218:324.e1–11. doi:10.1016/j.ajog.2017.12.007 pmid:29247637 [CrossRef] [PubMed] [Google Scholar]
25. Rodríguez MA, Afari N, Buchwald DS, National Institute of Diabetes and Digestive and Kidney Diseases Working Group on Urological Chronic Pelvic Pain. Evidence for overlap between urological and nonurological unexplained clinical conditions. *J Urol* 2009;182:2123–31. doi:10.1016/j.juro.2009.07.036 pmid:19758633 [CrossRef] [PubMed] [Web of Science] [Google Scholar]
26. Tirlapur SA, Kuhrt K, Chaliha C, et al. The 'evil twin syndrome' in chronic pelvic pain: A systematic review of prevalence studies of bladder pain syndrome and endometriosis. *Int J Surg* 2013;11:233–7. doi:10.1016/j.ijsu.2013.02.003 pmid:23419614 [CrossRef] [PubMed] [Google Scholar]
27. Chiaffarino F, Cipriani S, Ricci E, et al. Endometriosis and inflammatory bowel disease: A systematic review of the literature. *Eur J Obstet Gynecol Reprod Biol* 2020;252:246–51. doi:10.1016/j.ejogrb.2020.06.051 pmid:32629225 [CrossRef] [PubMed] [Google Scholar]
28. Singh SS, Missmer SA, Tu FF. Endometriosis and pelvic pain for the gastroenterologist. *Gastroenterol Clin North Am* 2022;51:195–211. doi:10.1016/j.gtc.2021.10.012 pmid:35135662 [CrossRef] [PubMed] [Google Scholar]
29. Farland LV, Degnan WJ 3rd., Bell ML, et al. Laparoscopically confirmed endometriosis and risk of incident stroke: A prospective cohort study. *Stroke* 2022;53:3116–22. doi:10.1161/STROKEAHA.122.039250 pmid:35861076 [CrossRef] [PubMed] [Google Scholar]
30. Mu F, Rich-Edwards J, Rimm EB, et al. Endometriosis and risk of coronary heart disease. *Circ Cardiovasc Qual Outcomes* 2016;9:257–64. doi:10.1161/CIRCOUTCOMES.115.002224 pmid:27025928 [Abstract/FREE Full Text] [Google Scholar]
31. Brawn J, Morotti M, Zondervan KT, et al. Central changes associated with chronic pelvic pain and endometriosis. *Hum Reprod Update* 2014;20:737–47. doi:10.1093/humupd/dmu025 pmid:24920437 [CrossRef] [PubMed] [Google Scholar]
32. Saraswat L, Avansina D, Cooper KG, et al. Risk of melanoma in women with endometriosis: A Scottish national cohort study. *Europ J Obstet Gynec Reprod Biol* doi:10.1016/j.ejogrb.2020.12.033
33. Yang F, Mortlock S, MacGregor S, et al. The International Endometriosis Genetics Consortium. Genetic relationship between endometriosis and

melanoma. *Front Reprod Health* 2021 Aug 2;3:711123. doi:10.3389/frph.2021.711123

34. O'malley J, Iacovou M, Holdsworth-Carson SJ. Evidence for an association between endometriosis and allergic and non-allergic food hypersensitivity is lacking. *Fron Reprod Health* 2021;3:726598. doi:10.3389/frph.2021.726598

35. Matalliotakis I, Cakmak H, Matalliotakis M, et al. High rate of allergies among women with endometriosis. *J Obstet Gynecol* 2012;32(3):291–3.

36. Antonio SL, Valentina Lucia LR, AgneseMaria CR, et al. Anxiety and depression in patients with endometriosis: Impact and management challenges. *Int J Womens Health* 2017;9:323–30. doi:10.2147/IJWH.S119729

37. Delanerolle G, Ramakrishnan R, Hapangama D, et al. A systematic review and meta-analysis of the endometriosis and mental-health sequelae; The ELEMI project. *Womens Health (Lond)* 2021;17:17455065211019717. Published online 2021 May 31. doi:10.1177/17455065211019717

38. Hansson GK. Inflammation, atherosclerosis, and coronary artery disease. *N Engl J Med* 2005;352:1685.

39. Santoro L, D'Onofrio F, Campo S, et al. Endothelial dysfunction but not increased carotid intima-media thickness in young European women with endometriosis. *Hum Reprod* 2012;27:1320.

40. Mu F, Rich-Edwards J, Rimm EB, et al. Endometriosis and risk of coronary heart disease. *Circ Cardiovasc Qual Outcome* 2016;9:257.

41. Pisanu A, Deplano D, Angioni S, et al. Rectal perforation from endometriosis in pregnancy case report and literature review. *World J Gastroenterol* 2010;16:648.

42. Brosens IA, Fusi L, Brosens JJ. Endometriosis is a risk factor for spontaneous hemo peritoneum during pregnancy. *Fertil Steril* 2009;92:1243.

43. Murphy SJ, Kaur A, Wullschleger ME. Endometrial decidualization: A rare cause of acute appendicitis during pregnancy. *J Surg Case Rep* 2016;2016.

44. Maggiore ULR, Ferrero S, Mangili G, et al. A systematic review on endometriosis during pregnancy: Diagnosis, misdiagnosis, complications and outcomes. *Hum Reprod Update* 2016;22:70.

45. Glavind MT, Forman A, Arendt LH, et al. Endometriosis and pregnancy complications: A Danish cohort study. *Fertil Steril* 2017;107:160.

46. Saraswat L, Ayansina DT, Cooper KG, et al. Pregnany outcomes in women with endometriosis: A national record linkage study. *BJOG* 2017;124:444.

47. Brosens IA, De Sutter P, Hamerlynck T, et al. Endometriosis is associated with a decreased risk of pre-eclampsia. *Hum Reprod* 2007;22:1725.

FURTHER READING

Horne AW, Missmer SA. Pathophysiology, diagnosis, and management of endometriosis. *BMJ* 2022;379 doi:10.1136/bmj-2022-070750 (Published 14 Nov 2022) Cite this as: *BMJ* 2022;379:e070750

The Women's Health Strategy: Ambitions Need Action to Improve Care for Endometriosis

....

Shalini Gadiyar

The health and wellbeing of women and girls over the course of their lives has long been neglected (1).

The Women's Health Strategy for England was published in July 2022. The Strategy resulted from a call for evidence, which received over 100,000 responses from the public, institutions, charities and researcher workers and over 400 written submissions from organizations and experts in health and care focusing on women's health priorities and gender health inequalities across England (2).

The key areas are summarized as ambitions in the strategy report (2): Ensuring women's voices are heard without stigma; improving women's access to medical services for female-specific illnesses as well as universal conditions such as dementia and stroke; and addressing intersectional disparities that affect women, such as age, ethnicity and disability, among many others. The strategy covers all gynaecological and obstetrical conditions including general health and wellbeing.

The government's ambition is to drive systemic changes so that the health needs of women and girls are better met. But it's the how, not the why, of this strategy that now needs detail, resources and accountability.

Although women make up 51% of the population and, on average, live longer than men, they spend a significantly greater proportion of their lives in ill health and disability when compared with men. Not enough focus is placed on women-specific issues like miscarriage or menopause, and women are under-represented when it comes to important clinical

DOI: 10.1201/9781032684819-23

trials. This has meant that not enough is known about conditions that only affect women like endometriosis.

This is a 10-year strategy that sets out a range of commitments to improve the health of women everywhere, including plans to increase female participation in research.

In the 2014 Chief Medical Officer's (Professor Dame Sally C Davies) annual report, the health of the 51% women (3) identified the widening disparities for girls and women during their adolescent, reproductive and post-reproductive years. The report's recommendations covered a range of areas including improving physical and mental health among mothers.

The issues raised then remain relevant today: for example, contraception service provision and help and support to improve mental health in women suffering with endometriosis. In some cases, health disparities have widened and been further exaggerated by the pandemic.

The Better for Women report (4) published in 2019 by the Royal College of Obstetricians and Gynaecologists (RCOG) highlighted the need to adopt a life-course approach, emphasizing the importance of preventative health interventions, instead of focusing on the treatment of established disease.

The executive summary and recommendations go on to recommend a life-course perspective, which offers potential for early intervention with the aim of reducing the progression. This includes, amongst others like cervical and breast cancer screening, earlier management of menstrual problems. Even though it does not specify endometriosis, early management of menstrual problems like painful periods is part of endometriosis care.

In the report, Dame Lesley Regan, immediate RCOG past-president (2016–2019) wrote: "To provide advice and care for girls and women across their life-course helps them to remain healthy and not just intervene when they experience problems." There is a requirement for better access to standardized, consistent information to allow women to make the decisions around their own health and wellbeing and a requirement to design health care services around the needs of women, very much needed for sufferers of endometriosis.

Regan, appointed as England's first Women's Health Ambassador (WHA) in June 2022, clearly stated:

When we get it right for women, everyone in our society benefits. This first Women's Health Strategy for England is the next step on the journey to reset the dial on women's health. The call for evidence, which informs the ambitions of the strategy, reiterates what I hear repeatedly from women: that our health care systems are failing them because NHS services are not designed to meet women's day-to-day needs.

All too often it forces women to navigate their way around multiple different health professionals and facilities trying to access basic services to maintain their health and wellbeing. The irony is that their care can easily be provided more conveniently and at significantly lower cost during a single visit to a women's health hub or centre if we adopt a "one-stop-shop" model. This strategy fits in nicely with endometriosis service provision.

(5)

Dame Lesley Regan said: "2022 was the year of the menopause, 2023 [should be] **menstrual-health awareness year.**"

"Make it just as common to talk about your period problems and knowing where to get help." This clearly means that women and girls should be empowered with information and knowledge about endometriosis and should seek early help from their GP.

The strategy acknowledges that organizations, particularly NHS England, National Institute for Health and Care Research (NIHR), NICE and Health Education England have substantial roles to play, but these roles, and accountability, are not explicitly delegated. Moreover, a timeline of 3 years for the first review of the strategy diminishes impetus to act promptly on delivery. This is especially relevant for initiatives such as endometriosis where despite NICE Guidelines, implementation has been delayed due to a deficit in funding and lack of priority for the organizations delivering care.

WHY DO WE NEED A WOMEN'S HEALTH STRATEGY?

While women in the UK, on average, live longer than men, they spend a significantly greater proportion of their lives in ill health and disability when compared with men (6). Historically the health and care system has been designed by men for men.

This "male as default" approach has been seen in:

- Research and clinical trials
- Education and training for health care professionals
- The design of health care policies and services

This has led to gaps in our data and evidence base that not enough is known about conditions that only affect women—for example, menopause or endometriosis. It has also resulted in inefficiencies in how services are delivered—for example, we know that many women have to move from service to service to have their reproductive health needs met.

VISION FOR WOMEN'S HEALTH STRATEGY FOR ENGLAND (7)

The key themes and areas of focus are:

- Women's voices must be heard
- Health care policies and services must be distributed
- Information and education is not only for the professionals but also the public
- Health in the workplace needs to be addressed
- Research, evidence and data should be distributed regularly

WOMEN'S HEALTH STRATEGY: PRIORITY AREAS (7)

In the call for evidence public survey, gynaecological conditions were the top topic that respondents picked for inclusion in the strategy, with 63% of respondents selecting this. Menstrual health was the fourth most selected topic, with 47% of respondents selecting this.

Access to information was a key issue, with only 8% of respondents feeling that they had access to enough information on gynaecological conditions, such as endometriosis and fibroids, and only 17% of respondents feeling that they had enough information on menstrual wellbeing.

There were concerns that women had not been listened to, for example, where pain is the main symptom—such as, being told that heavy and painful periods are "normal" or that the woman will "grow out of them." Women also said that they spoke to doctors on multiple occasions over many months or years before receiving a diagnosis for conditions such as endometriosis.

Gynaecological Conditions Included in the Strategy

- Heavy menstrual bleeding
- Premenstrual syndrome (PMS)
- Premenstrual dysphoric disorder (PMDD)
- **Endometriosis**
- Adenomyosis
- Fibroids
- Polycystic ovary syndrome (PCOS)

10-Year Ambitions of the Strategy (7)

- Women and girls are empowered to stay well throughout their lives, including through self-care. Women and girls should have an awareness of the different gynaecological conditions (such as endometriosis and PCOS) and less well-known conditions (such as adenomyosis), and an understanding of what a normal menstrual cycle should look like for them. Women and girls should know where, when and how to seek help for menstrual or gynaecological symptoms and what support and care they can expect

- All women and girls can access high-quality, personalized care within primary and community care, including access to contraception for the management of menstrual problems and gynaecological conditions. Where more specialist care is needed, women and girls can access diagnostic and treatment procedures in a timely manner

- *Women and girls with severe endometriosis experience better care where diagnosis time is reduced on the journey from initial GP appointment through to final diagnosis*

- Health care professionals in primary care are well-informed and trained in menstrual and gynaecological health and offer women and girls evidence-based advice and treatment

- NICE Guidelines for gynaecological conditions are developed where they do not currently exist and existing guidelines are updated rapidly in response to new evidence, and guidelines are implemented into practice. Guidelines are presented in an interactive format to support health care professionals to provide high-quality, cost-effective care

- Women and girls with menstrual and gynaecological conditions are supported to reach their full potential in education and the workplace. Education institutions and employers are well-equipped to support their students or workforce and are encouraged to implement evidence-based support such as workplace policies

WHAT ACTIONS ARE BEING TAKEN FOR ENDOMETRIOSIS

Regarding endometriosis, NHS England is updating the service specification for severe endometriosis in 2022 to 2023 (8). Service specifications are important for defining the standards of care expected from organizations commissioned by NHS England to provide specialist care. This update will ensure that specialist endometriosis services have access to the most up-to-date evidence and advice to improve standards of care for women with endometriosis.

HEALTH IN THE WORKPLACE: 10-YEAR AMBITIONS OF WHS

Women's health concerns are often overlooked by employers. But with vast female workforces, employers need to be more supportive and proactive on women's health.

The WHS includes an investment of £1.97 million in workplace support initiatives for women. Access to good occupational health services, mental health support, line manager training and workplace adjustments are perceived to be ways to create a working environment that is conducive to managing a health condition or maintaining good health at work—in addition to tackling stigmas and taboos around menstruation, menopause and gynaecological conditions—so that women feel able to speak up and access support (9).

The British Standards Institution finds *almost a third of women leave the workforce before retirement age due to health*, which can culminate in huge cost implications for employers. It's time for employers to take steps to ensure that female workers are supported, have choices, are treated with compassion and are able to continue working wherever possible.

In the written submissions, organizations recommended employers introduce or improve their workplace provisions and policies to better support women in different situations. This included:

- Helping women to manage the impact of symptoms of menstrual health problems, conditions such as endometriosis or menopause in the workplace
- Supporting women and partners undergoing fertility treatment or who have experienced a pregnancy loss which can happen in women with endometriosis
- Allowing women to discuss health issues openly
- Improving managers' and employers' understanding of symptoms

EDUCATION AND TRAINING: 10-YEAR AMBITIONS OF WHS

NICE Guidelines

The National Institute of Health and Care Excellence (NICE) provides authoritative, evidence-based guidelines for health care professionals on best practice. Guidelines are developed by experts based on a thorough assessment of the available evidence and through extensive engagement with stakeholders. NICE Guidelines are often the first port of call for health care professionals, and it is vital that they reflect the most up-to-date evidence.

NICE has agreed to update the guideline on endometriosis diagnosis and management.

Its review will cover three areas for improvement:

- Diagnosis including the use of imaging
- Surgical management
- Surgical management where fertility is a priority

NICE undertook a surveillance review that led to this decision, and that review also highlighted gaps in research and evidence including recognizing the need for more research into pain management, mental wellbeing and endometriosis outside the pelvis, such as thoracic endometriosis. It's good to see NICE's commitment to explore new—and much needed—research opportunities on these topics with the National Institute for Health Research (NIHR), the government research funding body.

This is a positive development and the new guidelines on endometriosis's diagnosis and management are published on 11 November 2024.

The NICE Strategy 2021 to 2026 (10) ensures that guidelines are easily implemented and accessible to health care professionals, as well as commissioners of local services, to improve the care of patients with endometriosis.

Best Practice Resources for Health Care Professionals

Professional bodies and other organizations have developed evidence-based resources and materials to support health care professionals to translate guidance into delivery of care.

The RCGP has developed a women's health toolkit (11) that aims to support practising GPs. This resource is continually updated to ensure GPs have the most up-to-date advice to provide the best care for their patients. Within this, RCGP has worked in partnership with Endometriosis UK to develop a menstrual wellbeing toolkit (12) for GPs and other health care professionals.

The Primary Care Women's Health Forum (PCWHF) also produces training materials to bring guidance into practice for primary care in a range of formats. This covers a range of women's health issues including the menopause, endometriosis and menstrual disorders.

ACCESS TO SERVICE (13)

Ambitions are:

- Women and girls can access services that meet their needs across the entire span of their life-course—from adolescence through the middle and reproductive years to menopause and the post-reproductive era, including for general health conditions and disabilities. These needs must be met at one time and at one place, by developing local pathways that improves access to services—for example, women's health hubs
- *There are clear pathways between primary, community and secondary care settings delivered, for example, through the expansion of community diagnostic centres and surgical hubs, and women and girls can access secondary care and specialist services for conditions such as endometriosis when needed.* Achieving this ambition will require partnership working across all policy, commissioning and delivery partners

RESEARCH AND EVIDENCE (14)

High-quality research that represents a range of women and health issues is vital for evidence-based policy-making and clinical decisions.

In September 2021, the findings of **a study exploring what happens in primary care when women present with endometriosis-like symptoms** (15) were published. These findings will be used to understand the barriers to diagnosing endometriosis.

We are taking action and encouraging high-quality research through the NIHR (the nation's largest funder of health and care research, which spends £1 billion from the Department of Health and Social Care budget on research every year) and UKRI (a national funding agency investing nearly £8 billion a year in research and innovation in the UK and internationally, sponsored by the Department for Business, Energy and Industrial Strategy). Within UKRI, the Medical Research Council (MRC) funds the highest volume of research relevant to women's health.

(14)

The NIHR has made significant investments into research on a wide range of women's health conditions, including gynaecological conditions, pregnancy and menopause. This includes a £2 million randomized control trial on endometriosis to examine the effectiveness of surgery compared with non-surgical interventions to manage chronic pelvic pain in women.

EXPECT Centre for Endometriosis is advancing research into endometriosis and its management.

To make the strategy a reality, there need to be clearly defined areas of responsibility for data, research, health care, public health and school education in women's health. Routinely collected data, quality assured, and as near to real-time as possible should be used to monitor access to, and uptake of, key services by population groups.

The service delivery to patients with endometriosis could be evaluated using data on delayed diagnosis, (refer to Chapter 12), what investigations to do and whether they were done (refer to Chapter 6), timely referral to appropriate service providers, timely referral to specialist endometriosis centre (refer to Chapter 11), and addressing endometriosis-associated infertility (refer to Chapter 15). There should be a national approach to women's health data, mandating reporting of all research and audits by sex and gender.

An annual review of research, such as the Research and Development (RAND) analysis of spend on endometriosis would improve transparency.

QUALITY OF CARE

Quality of care is a multidimensional concept that is affected by stakeholders' priorities and context (16). Attributes of quality of care include access to care, effectiveness of care, safety, equitability, communication, acceptability, efficiency and privacy and confidentiality (16).

Women's health services, particularly sexual and reproductive health services, are often not provided at a level of quality that meets human rights standards (17,18).

> *With reference to endometriosis, multidimensions of accountability are needed by adopting a framework built on three pillars: Monitoring, review of care provided and action taken to improve the service. There should be independent verification with clear recommendation for changes: for example, delay in referral or delay in laparoscopy to make a diagnosis. Participatory monitoring and accountability mechanisms that meaningfully engage women at the sub-national, national and global levels are a critical part of this.*

ENDOMETRIOSIS AND COVID-19

Endometriosis patients were undeniably impacted by the COVID-19 pandemic, which caused the worsening of symptoms, such as dysmenorrhea, pelvic pain, anxiety, depression and fatigue.

Disruption in hormonal and immunological processes which may occur in endometriosis may increase susceptibility to SARS-CoV-2 infection. A systematic review and meta-analysis of 474 articles was done. A total of 17,799 patients were analyzed. The pooled prevalence of SARS-CoV-2 infection in endometriosis patients was 7.5%. Pooled estimates for the health impacts were 47.2% for decreased access to medical care, 49.3% increase in dysmenorrhea, 75% increase in anxiety, 59.4% increase in depression, and 68.9% increase in fatigue (19).

The prevalence of SARS-CoV-2 infection in endometriosis patients was substantial. Undeniably, endometriosis patients were negatively impacted regarding access to medical care during the COVID-19 pandemic. Moreover, a majority of patients experienced the worsening of pelvic pain, anxiety, depression and fatigue, whereas approximately half of the patients reported increased dysmenorrhea, dyspareunia and dyschezia (20).

Delivery Plan for Tackling the COVID-19 Backlog of Care (21)

Published in February 2022, this plan to address the COVID-19 backlog of care sets out strategies to reduce waiting times and improve patient experience across all specialty areas, including gynaecology and urogynaecology. This includes plans to:

- Communicate better with patients about treatment options and establish a network for people waiting a long time, including through the *My Planned Care* patient platform
- Roll out up to 160 community diagnostic centres across the country to help clear backlogs of people waiting for clinical tests, many for gynaecological pathways—for example, ultrasound scanning, blood tests and hysteroscopy to investigate heavy menstrual bleeding
- Roll-out surgical hubs across the country

Focusing on care provision of endometriosis patients means communication with patients about treatment options available, getting early ultrasound scans done and, most important, early hysteroscopy and histology, which are the diagnostic tools of endometriosis.

KEY POINT SUMMARY

- Menstrual health and gynaecological conditions including endometriosis are recognized among the priority areas to be addressed in the Women's Health Strategy.
- The 10-year ambition of the strategy includes measures to reduce lengthy diagnosis times, improve care for those with endometriosis, and provide more support for health care professionals and increased funding for research.
- Women and girls with severe endometriosis experience better care where diagnosis time is reduced on the journey from initial GP appointment through to final diagnosis.
- NICE undertook a surveillance review that led to this decision and that review also highlighted gaps in research and evidence including recognizing the need for more research into pain management, mental wellbeing and endometriosis outside the pelvis, such as thoracic endometriosis.
- Employers are to introduce and improve their workplace provisions and policies to better support women suffering with menstrual health problems and conditions like endometriosis.

REFERENCES

1. Department of Health and Social Care. *Policy paper: Our vision for the Women's Health Strategy for England.* 2021. www.gov.uk/government/publications/our-vision-for-the-womens-health-strategy-for-england/our-vision-for-the-womens-health-strategy-for-england.
2. Womersley K, Hockham C, Mullins E. The Women's Health Strategy: Ambitions need action and accountability. *BMJ* 2022;378. doi:10.1136/bmj.o2059 (Published 19 Aug 2022) Cite this as: *BMJ* 2022;378:o2059
3. *The health of the 51%: Women report Cameron years (2015–2016). Public Health 11 December 2015.* www.gov.uk/government/publication/.
4. *Better for women report by RCOG: Primary Care Women's Health Forum.* www.rcog.org.uk/better-for-women/.
5. GOV.UK. *Women's Health Strategy for England.* www.gov.uk/womens-health-strategy.
6. *Health state life expectancies, UK: 2018 to 2020.* www.ons.gov.uk/peoplepopulationandcommunity/healthandsocialcare/healthandlifeexpectancies/bullietins/healthsatelifeexpectancieuk/2018to2020.
7. *Our vision for the Women's Health Strategy for England.* 2021 Dec 23 www.gov.uk/government/publications.
8. NHS England. *Service specification.* www.england.nhs.uk/commissioning/spec-services/npc-crg/group-e/e09.
9. GOV.UK. *Women's health strategy for England.* www.gov.uk/government/publications/womens-health-strategy-for-england/womens-health-strategy-for-england#health-in-the-workplace.
10. National Institute for Health and Care Excellence. *NICE strategy 2021 to 2026.* https://www.nice.org.uk/about/who-we-are/corporate-publications/the-nice-strategy-2021-to-2026.

11. RCGP Learning. *Women's health toolkit—Royal College of General Practitioners—Online learning environment.* https://elearning.rcgp.org.uk.
12. RCGP Learning. *Women's health toolkit: Menstrual health.* https://elearning.rcgp.org.uk.
13. GOV.UK. *Women's health strategy for England.* www.gov.uk/government/publications/womens-health-strategy-for-england/womens-health-strategy-for-england#access-to-services.
14. GOV.UK. *Policy paper: Women health strategy for England.* www.gov.uk/government/publications/womens-health-strategy-for-england (updated 30 Aug 2022).
15. Dixon S, McNiven A, Talbot A, et al. Navigating possible endometriosis in primary care: A qualitative study of GP perspectives. *Br J Gen Pract* 2021;71(710):e668–76. doi:10.3399/BJGP.2021.0030
16. Bruce J. Fundamental elements of the quality of care: A simple framework. *Stud Fam Plan* 1990;21:61–91.
17. Germain A. Meeting Human Rights Norms for the Quality of Sexual and Reproductive Health Information and Services: Discussion Paper: ICPD beyond 2014. International Conference on Human Rights. 2013.
18. Independent Expert Review Group (iERG). Every woman, every child: Strengthening equity and dignity through health: The second report of the independent Expert Review Group (iERG) in information and accountability for women's and children's health. WHO, 2013.
19. Kabani Z, Ramos-Nino ME, Ramdass PVAK. Endometriosis and COVID-19: A systematic review and meta-analysis. *Int J Mol Sci* 26 Oct 2022;23(21):12951. doi:10.3390/ijms232112951 pmid:36361745 pmcid:PMC9657778
20. Ashkenazi MS, Huseby OL, Kroken G, et al. COVID-19 pandemic and the consequential effect on patients with endometriosis. *Hum Reprod Open* 2022 Mar 18;2022(2):hoac013. doi:10.1093/hropen/hoac013.eCollection 2022
21. *Delivery plan for tackling the COVID-19 backlog of elective care.* www.england.nhs.uk/coronavirus/publication.

FURTHER READING

www.rcog.org.uk/better-for-women/
www.gov.uk/womens-health-strategy

CHAPTER 18

Education in Schools: Menstrual Health and Raising Awareness

....

Margaret Heywood

No young girl should have to suffer in silence thinking that having very painful period is normal, especially when it is an issue affecting their daily lives.

Menstruation education is an essential part of wider menstrual literacy. Some girls with endometriosis experience debilitating endometriosis-associated pain that prevents them from going to school.

Menstrual stigma and shame can contribute to barriers to learning.

Addressing endometriosis can reduce school absenteeism. Girls need some support rather than dismissive teachers who do not believe or understand this condition and just think she is having painful periods and it is all normal.

Menstrual health education programs can address poor attendance, poor performance and lack of participation in school activities and friends making fun!

Menstrual morbidity plays a significant role in adolescent females' lives. There are no studies to date reporting such data from menstrual health education programs in schools.

There has never been a need to integrate menstrual learning within all curriculum areas across school life. Why do we not have an educational program in schools aiming for early recognition of symptoms when there is enough evidence that 1 in 10 women suffer from endometriosis and that it takes 8 years to make a diagnosis. One factor of lengthy delay in diagnosis is poor education and not talking about menstrual health.

Consistent delivery of a menstrual health education program in schools can increase awareness of endometriosis.

DOI: 10.1201/9781032684819-24

MENSTRUATION

The onset of menstruation can be confusing or even alarming for girls if they are not prepared. Pupils should be taught key facts about the menstrual cycle including what is an average period, range of menstrual products and the implications for emotional and physical health. In addition to curriculum content, schools should also make adequate and sensitive arrangements to help girls prepare for and manage menstruation including with requests for menstrual products. Schools will need to consider the needs of their cohort of pupils in designing this content (1).

Menstrual Health

The term "menstrual health" has seen increased use across advocacy, programming, policy and research, but it has lacked a consistent, self-contained definition (2).

As a rapidly growing field of research and practice, a comprehensive definition is needed to ensure menstrual health is prioritized as a unified objective in global health, development and national policy and funding frameworks elucidate the breadth of menstrual health, even where different needs may be prioritized in different sectors, facilitating a shared vocabulary through which stakeholders can communicate across silos to share learning.

Menstrual health is a state of complete physical, mental and social wellbeing and not merely the absence of disease or infirmity in relation to the menstrual cycle.

Achieving menstrual health implies that women, girls and all other people who experience a menstrual cycle, throughout their life-course, can:

- Access accurate, timely, age-appropriate information about the menstrual cycle, menstruation and changes experienced throughout the life-course, as well as related self-care and hygiene practices

- Care for their bodies during menstruation such that their preferences, hygiene, comfort, privacy and safety are supported. This includes accessing and using effective and affordable menstrual materials and having supportive facilities and services, including water, sanitation and hygiene services, for washing the body and hands, changing menstrual materials and cleaning and/or disposing of used materials

- Access timely diagnosis, treatment and care for menstrual cycle–related discomforts and disorders, including access to appropriate health services and resources, pain relief and strategies for self-care

- Experience a positive and respectful environment in relation to the menstrual cycle, free from stigma and psychological distress, including the resources and support they need to confidently care for their bodies and make informed decisions about self-care throughout their menstrual cycle

- Decide whether and how to participate in all spheres of life, including civil, cultural, economic, social and political, during all phases of the menstrual cycle, free from menstrual-related exclusion, restriction, discrimination, coercion and/or violence

A New Zealand model examining the impact of an education program in schools on early recognition of symptoms suggesting endometriosis showed strong evidence that consistent delivery of a menstrual health education program in schools increases adolescent student awareness of endometriosis (3).

In addition, there is suggestive evidence that in a geographical area of consistent delivery of the program, a shift in earlier presentation of young women to a specialized health service is observed.

In a region of consistent delivery of the education program, student awareness of endometriosis was 32% in 2015. Overall, in 2015, 13% of students experienced distressing menstrual symptoms and 27% of students sometimes or always missed school due to menstrual symptoms. Further, in one region of consistent delivery of the menstrual health education program, data show an increase in younger patients attending for specialized endometriosis care (3).

Menstrual cycle education in UK schools is inconsistent and inadequate, and teachers feel they lack time, confidence and subject knowledge, according to new research involving Nottingham Trent University (4).

Researchers conducted a survey of 789 UK primary and secondary school teachers, 88% of whom felt that periods affected pupils' attendance, participation in exercise, behaviour and confidence (4).

The study, led by Swansea University, found that only 53% of secondary school teachers reported that menstrual cycle education lessons were taught in their school. Of the teachers who were aware of their school's menstrual cycle syllabus across primary and secondary schools, 144 reported that a maximum of two lessons were provided within one academic year.

Ninety percent of teachers who responded to the survey were female, and almost 1 in 4 (23%) reported that they were uncomfortable teaching about the menstrual cycle, with many drawing on their own experiences, and less than half felt confident in their knowledge. The report concluded that:

> *this is such an important area to be addressed to enable young girls to have a sound understanding of their menstrual cycles. We hope that this research highlights some of the gaps in areas of education and enables future education guidance to be more consistent across all schools.*
>
> (4)

This study calls for improvements to be made to menstrual cycle education for boys and girls across the UK, including:

- Making time available for delivery, particularly to increase the regularity of teaching and lowering the age at which young people are first taught
- Delivering resources for teachers to deliver information relating to emotional, social and physical aspects of the menstrual cycle
- Providing training support to teachers, with the minimum expectation for teachers to receive online professional development through e-learning and/or webinar

According to Endometriosis UK; menstrual wellbeing education was made compulsory in Wales in late December 2021, and wellbeing education began to be taught in primary and secondary schools in England in September 2020. The education should focus on what is a normal menstrual cycle and how and where to seek help (5).

For too long, young people have not been given the tools and the education they need to make informed choices about their health. It takes an average of 8 years to get a diagnosis of endometriosis in the UK and symptoms can start in puberty, meaning some children and teenagers suffer with potentially debilitating symptoms for the majority of their school life. Without learning about menstrual wellbeing in school, young people will continue to suffer in silence (5).

A survey done in 2022 on teachers' perceptions and experiences of menstrual cycle education and support in UK schools (6) captured information on menstrual education in schools, teacher's knowledge and confidence of the menstrual cycle, support provided to teachers, provision of menstrual products in school and perceived impact of the menstrual cycle on young people in school.

The 498 teachers in the study reported lessons were provided on the menstrual cycle (63%), predominantly delivered within personal, social, health and economic or science subjects, with over half of the lessons focusing on the biology (56%) or provision of menstrual products (40%) rather than lived experiences (14%). Teachers perceived the menstrual cycle affected participation in PE (88%), pupil confidence (88%), school attendance (82%) and attitude and behaviour (82%).

Overall, 80% of teachers felt receiving training would be beneficial to improve menstrual education. The results highlight education is scientifically focused, with less education on management of symptoms or lived experiences. Teachers also perceive the menstrual cycle to influence multiple aspects of school attendance and personal performance.

> *There is a need to address menstrual education provided in schools across the UK to help empower girls to manage their menstrual cycle, preventing a negative impact on health and school performance* (6).

Relationships Education, Relationships and Sex Education (RSE) and Health Education statutory guidance for England, published in 2019 and updated in 2021, includes very brief mentions of menstruation in the curriculum (7).

The guidance mentions covering puberty including menstruation in health education and that it should, as far as possible, be addressed before onset.

Pupils should be taught key facts about the menstrual cycle including what is an average period, range of menstrual products and the implications for emotional and physical health. Schools will need to consider the needs of their cohort of pupils in designing this content (7).

A new curriculum model is necessary to support teachers in planning lessons that will grow with young people and meet their learning needs appropriately at each age and stage because, despite more awareness, there is no joined up, practical strategy focusing on painful periods.

A new policy paper on the Women's Health Strategy for England declares the following aims and sets these as 10-year ambitions (8):

- Girls and boys receive high-quality, evidence-based education on menstrual and gynaecological health from an early age
- Across the population, there is increased awareness, and menstrual health and gynaecological conditions are no longer taboo subjects in any aspect of society
- Women and girls are empowered to stay well throughout their lives, including through self-care

- Women and girls have an awareness of the different gynaecological conditions (such as endometriosis and PCOS) and less well-known conditions (such as adenomyosis) and an understanding of what a normal menstrual cycle should look like for them
- Women and girls know where, when and how to seek help for menstrual or gynaecological symptoms and what support and care they can expect

Early engagement with menstrual health education, from the first interactions with sexual health education in school, should set the stage for later life. This education should provide an overview of the signs and symptoms of menstrual abnormalities which can be recognized, communicated and managed early. For example, teaching that severe period pain or heavy bleeding is abnormal may accelerate diagnosis and access to appropriate care for a menstrual-related condition (9).

> *Inadequate menstrual health education in the UK contributes to delayed and poor treatment for menstrual-related disorders, such as endometriosis and uterine fibroids, many of which severely impact quality of life.*

The current deficiency in quality menstrual education leads to confusion, inaccurate beliefs and negative views on menstruation and related conditions. There is a lack of understanding of what constitutes menstrual dysfunction and *when, where and how* to seek care. Improvement can only be achieved by better education of the clinical characteristics of endometriosis, not only among general practitioners but also school nurses, who play crucial roles in early diagnosis. This is achievable through menstrual education programs that incorporate the disease as a leading cause of pain. Emphasizing appropriate, cross-collaborative strategies to optimize outcomes can transform endometriosis care and reduce the role of "menstrual silence" in its diagnosis and treatment (10).

Embarking on robust educational programs that begin in the primary setting and are shared across varied resources will enhance literacy on painful menstruation, thereby affording access to better, earlier care and improving the quality of life. By revitalizing menstrual communication and key conversations, we can put an end to the secrecy, silence, shame and pain (10).

There is a need for menstrual education in schools, with the topic being offered even before menarche in order to better prepare girls for the experience and continuing throughout their educational career so that students can build upon their basic knowledge of the many themes involved with menstrual health (11). A three-pronged approach has been suggested (12) to better inform individuals about dysmenorrhea specifically: Having the school nurse provide educational leaflets to increase familiarity with the condition; encouraging health professionals to be more proactive in asking patients about the topic so that young menstruators with dysmenorrhea may be more likely to disclose their pain and symptoms; and finally, joint promotion by health professionals and schools of reliable, authoritative websites and resources for additional guidance.

Evidence demonstrates that consistent delivery of a menstrual health education program in schools specifically increases awareness of endometriosis (13). One successful example of such program is School Nurse Initiative (14). The goal is to provide a toolkit to school nurses to help educate their students and the school community about the disease. School nurses play a crucial role in recognizing early signs of the disease in their students and can provide critical information about endometriosis along with important resources.

Guided by preliminary results of the ongoing Black Women's Reproductive Health (BWRH) project (15), the key recommendation to support Black women's menstrual and reproductive health is mandatory training for health care professionals and those who teach about menstrual health in schools, covering the historical development of current menstrual health knowledge and attitudes and the pervasive impact on those who menstruate, with particular focus on racially marginalized populations (9).

Period Positive (16) is committed to working with young people and communities, challenging and pushing the menstrual discourse forward so that it is in line with reproductive justice, social justice and human rights values of equity, inclusivity and sustainability. Some of the pledges are—"Study up on the biology of menstruation and reproductive health so that you understand how hormones and glands help the organs in your body to function healthily and so you can recognize if things are going wrong," "Fight for the rights of people whose menstruation causes extra problems because they are facing unfairness or discrimination in another part of their lives" and "Remember that no one thing will make it easier for people to manage menstruation. It's a combination of education about biology, understanding negative messages, awareness of different products, choice, availability and taboo breaking—all working together."

High-quality, timely and taboo-free menstrual education is vital. A Period Positive National Curriculum can build the foundations of knowledge in this important area of health.

KEY POINT SUMMARY

- There is a need to address menstrual education provided in schools across the UK to help empower girls to manage their menstrual cycle, preventing a negative impact on health and school performance.
- There is strong suggestive evidence that consistent delivery of a menstrual health education program in schools increases adolescent student awareness of endometriosis.
- It's integral that teachers are supported to improve their confidence and knowledge of the menstrual cycle for young people—both boys and girls. It should no longer be a taboo subject. We need to reframe the narrative and normalize conversations about menstruation.
- We still have a long way to go when it comes to period education across the UK. We face the danger of disadvantaging girls by failing to help them prepare, manage and understand physical and emotional symptoms when menstruating.
- Adopt the Period Positive National Curriculum, a framework that gives a list of suggestions for being fair, respectful and inclusive while we learn and grow our menstrual literacy. It is evidence-based, comprehensive and inclusive.

REFERENCES

1. *Physical health and mental wellbeing (Primary and secondary).* www.gov.uk/government/publications (accessed 13 Sep 2021).
2. Hennegan J, Winkler IT, Bobel C, et al. Menstrual health: A definition for policy, practice, and research. *Sex Reprod Health Matters* 2021;29(1):1911618.
3. Bush D, Brick E, East NC, et al. Affiliations expand. *Aust N Z J Obstet Gynaecol* 2017 Aug 57(4):452–7. Endometriosis education in schools: A New Zealand model examining the impact of an education program in schools on early recognition of symptoms suggesting endometriosis.
4. *Insufficient menstrual cycle education provided in UK schools, study finds.* www.ntu.ac.uk.about-us.news
5. *Endometriosis UK.* www.endometriosis-uk.org/information
6. Brown N, Williams R, Bruinvels G, Piasecki J, Forrest L J. Teachers' perceptions and experiences of menstrual cycle education and support in UK schools. pmid:35237766, PMCID: PMC8882726, DOI: 10.3389/fgwh.2022.827365
7. *Relationships and sex education (RSE) and health education.* www.gov.uk/government/publications
8. *Women's Health Strategy for England—GOV.UK.* www.gov.uk/government/publications.

9. Perro D, Seglah H, Abrahams V, et al. Black women's menstrual and reproductive health: A critical call for action in the UK. *BMJ* 2022;379. doi:10.1136/bmj.o3052 (Published 22 Dec 2022) Cite this as: *BMJ* 2022; 379:o3052

10. Guidone, HC. The womb wanders not: Enhancing endometriosis education in a culture of menstrual misinformation, Chapter 22. In Bobel C, et al. *The Palgrave Handbook of Critical Menstruation Studies. Heather C guidone.* www.ncbi.nlm.nih.gov/books/NBK565622

11. Cooper SC, Koch PB. "Nobody told me nothin": Communication about menstruation among low-income African-American women. *Women & Health* 2007;46(1):57–78. [PubMed]

12. Subasinghe AK, Happo L, Jayasinghe YL, et al. Prevalence and severity of dysmenorrhoea, and management options reported by young Australian women. *Aust Fam Physician* 2016 Nov;45(11):829–34. [PubMed]

13. Bush D, Brick E, East MC, et al. Endometriosis education in schools: A New Zealand model examining the impact of an education program in schools on early recognition of symptoms suggesting endometriosis. *Aust N Z J Obstet Gynaecol* 2017 Aug;57(4):452–7. [PubMed]

14. *The endo what? Documentary team school nurse initiative.* www.endowhat. com/school-nurse-initiative

15. Abrahams V, Perro D, Seglah HA, et al. *Black Women's Reproductive Health: Project Report. T.A.P. Project.* 2022. https://tapproject.co.uk/wp-content/uploads/2022/08/a40c0490-2880-4ffc-b231-386415f0bd3f.pdf

16. Quint C. *A Period Positive National Curriculum for England.* https:// period-positive-menstruation/wp-content/uploads/2022/07/a-period-positive-national-curriculum-chella-quint-20-july-2022.pdf (accessed 20 July 2022).

FURTHER READING

Women's Health Strategy for England—GOV.UK. www.gov.uk/government/ publications

Endometriosis UK. www.endometriosis-uk.org/information

CHAPTER 19

Advances in Endometriosis Research: From Bench to Bedside

....

*Deborah P. Fischer, Catherine E.W. Pennington,
Cohen J. Loveder and Kay M. Marshall*

Endometriosis has gained recognition as a debilitating chronic disorder that has a major impact not only on patients' physical health but also on their work, daily life, relationships and mental health, in addition to the wider economy. The burden is worsened by the reliance on surgical diagnosis and hormonal treatments that prevent pregnancy and carry side effects.

Slow progress in changing the landscape for women's health may be a result of the "male as default" approach to medical research and a lack of funding disproportionate to disease prevalence and severity (1,2). Endometriosis still only constitutes a fraction of the health budget in the USA 0.038% (3) and UK 0.02% (4), despite it affecting an estimated 190 million women of reproductive age worldwide (5). This gender disparity has now been recognized, and the available funding and number of researchers are gradually increasing to fill our knowledge gaps. As awareness of endometriosis grows and discussions are had, researchers aim to provide innovations in diagnostic and treatment strategies, moving from bench to bedside.

WHAT IS THE FUTURE OF DIAGNOSTICS?

It can be extremely difficult to diagnose endometriosis, taking 8 years 10 months on average after symptom onset in the UK, with other countries suffering longer delays (6). This can be attributed to multiple factors, including the lack of definitive, inexpensive and non-invasive tests.

DOI: 10.1201/9781032684819-25

The commercialization of such a diagnostic tool would help to treat patients earlier in disease progression. This would not only improve their quality of life but reduce the economic burden of endometriosis, which is estimated to cost the UK alone £8.2 billion per year in treatment, loss of work and health care costs (7).

WHAT ABOUT IMAGING MODALITIES?

Transvaginal ultrasound and magnetic resonance imaging (MRI) can be useful tools when investigating suspected endometriosis, especially endometriomas. Imaging for deep-infiltrating endometriosis (DIE), however, is only clear in certain anatomical locations, such as the pouch of Douglas (POD), and is suitable as a triage test (8,9) (Table 19.1). Because superficial endometriosis (SE) can be small and discrete, these imaging modalities cannot rule out the diagnosis (8). Improvements in the application of these tools are being continually investigated to compensate for this limitation. Chapron et al. (2019) suggested that laparoscopic diagnosis should no longer be favoured over the use of thorough interviews to identify high-risk patients followed by imaging to confirm the disease (10).

A recently completed phase-II study sponsored by the University of North Carolina evaluated 18F-fluoroestradiol PET positron emission tomography (PET) combined with MRI as a diagnostic tool for endometriosis (8). 18F-fluoroestradiol PET binds to oestrogen receptors, highlighting their heightened expression in endometrial lesions. However, the combined techniques still lacked sensitivity (ability to detect disease presence) and specificity (measure of false positive diagnosis). Only six control patients were enrolled in this study, which limits what can be inferred (11).

Another clinical trial sponsored by McMaster University is using ultrasound and molecular biomarkers in combination to accurately diagnose SE. This novel technique is named SonoPODography and requires cervically injected saline to accumulate in the pouch of Douglas (POD), which can then be visualized in more detail with ultrasound. The injected saline would then be aspirated and tested for various biomarkers (12). If reliable, this technique would offer value for detection of superficial lesions found in the POD. Theoretically, combining ultrasound with confirmed biomarkers for endometriosis would give greater diagnostic ability; the results of this pilot study and proprietary biomarkers are yet to be seen.

Indocyanine green (ICG) fluorescence imaging has also recently been adopted to enhance intraoperative detection of endometriosis. ICG

TABLE 19.1 Diagnostic Imaging Tools for Endometriosis and Their Characteristics

Imaging	Benefits	Limitations	Sensitivity	Specificity	Reference
MRI	Non-invasive Can detect endometriomas	No reliable detection of SE, expensive	Endometriomas: 95% DIE: 94%	Endometriomas: 91% DIE: 77%	(8)
SonoPODography	Reliable detection of SE	More invasive than imaging alone due to saline injection	Unknown	Unknown	(12)
18F-Fluoroestradiol PET/MRI	Specific lesion detection via targeting oestrogen receptors	More expensive and poorer image resolution than MRI alone; limited studies to support use	67%	NA due to limited sample size	(11)
Transvaginal ultrasound	Non-invasive More cost-effective than MRI and surgery Can detect endometriomas	Cannot reliably detect SE	Endometriomas: 93% DIE: 79%	Endometriomas: 96% DIE: 94%	(8)
Near-infrared ICG-augmented surgery	Fluorescence-guided resection of DIE and vascular organs	Lack of randomized controlled trials to support use over white light imaging	DIE: 82%	DIE: 97.9%	(14)

rapidly binds to proteins confined to the blood and lymphatic systems, enabling distinction between healthy tissues, hyper-vascularized areas and fibrotic endometriotic nodules under near-infrared light. This has been promising for the evaluation of bowel anastomoses and ureterolysis post-surgery (13). However, there is no clear consensus for its usefulness in ICG-augmented endometriosis surgery, which is still under evaluation.

THE SEARCH FOR NEW BIOMARKERS

Ongoing research to identify biomarkers is focusing on a multitude of inflammatory cytokines that relate to the increased numbers of peritoneal macrophages and their target products in endometriosis (15). However, whether this inflammation is causal or merely a downstream result of disease pathology is unknown. One study showed that the inflammatory cytokines interleukin (IL)-1β, IL-6, and tumour necrosis factor (TNF)α caused aberrant signalling in eutopic endometrial cells from women with endometriosis but not from those without (16). Later work identified these same three cytokines as being upregulated in the serum of 80 women with endometriosis, compared to 80 healthy controls (15). IL-1β and IL-6 were analyzed to validate this prediction, which gave a specificity of 85% and 95%, respectively. This means that approximately 15% and 5% of individuals diagnosed with endometriosis would receive a false positive diagnosis, respectively. Both cytokines also lacked sensitivity (<60%); therefore, almost half of patients with the disease would not be diagnosed with endometriosis using this technique. Later research confirmed that the expression of these cytokines was not significantly different between patients with endometriosis and those with other benign gynaecological conditions (17). Nevertheless, cancer antigen 125 (CA125) levels were significantly higher in endometriosis patients. Others have found similar results (18), suggesting that serum CA125 positively correlates with pathological characteristics of endometriosis (19). Unfortunately, the specificity and sensitivity of CA125 as a biomarker for endometriosis is lacking, in part due to the involvement of CA125 in ovarian cancer (20), endometrial cancer (21) and other diseases (22). Additionally, lifestyle choices, menstruation and ethnicity can all influence the serum concentration of CA125 (20).

This highlights a common issue with the use of inflammatory cytokines as biomarkers for endometriosis. Cytokines tend to also be upregulated in patients with other disorders, including diabetes (23,24), polycystic ovaries (25,26) and irritable bowel syndrome (27), the latter of which has overlapping symptoms with endometriosis. Comorbidities common with endometriosis may also increase systemic levels of inflammatory cytokines (28).

Overall, systemic cytokines alone are unlikely to provide the specificity required of a reliable diagnostic tool. However, they may be useful as an adjunct to imaging, to monitor pathogenesis, therapeutic response and recurrence of endometriosis. Furthermore, sampling cytokines from a source local to lesion sites may provide more specific analysis of the extra-uterine environment of interest (29).

WHICH BIOFLUID IS BEST FOR BIOMARKER RESEARCH?

Much clinical research utilizes serum as a source of biomarkers. Menstrual effluent may provide more insightful and specific indicators of endometriosis, especially since it contains endometrial cells that can be tested for specific genes or protein markers. Endometrial cells can also be cultured from the non-invasive collection of menstrual fluid (30). Recent research showed that menstrual effluent from women with endometriosis lacks a specific population of proliferative natural killer cells compared to those without clinical symptoms (31). This work has led to clinical trials pursuing menstrual effluent as a source of biomarkers to screen for endometriosis and to advise which individuals should be prioritized for laparoscopic diagnosis (32).

Saliva is another potential diagnostic fluid. Bendifallah et al. (2022) analyzed saliva from 200 women with chronic pelvic pain in search of suitable endometriosis biomarkers. Profiling microRNA expression identified 2,561 transcripts, 109 of which showed an endometriosis signature when an algorithm was used (33). This group has more recently released interim data from a multicentre study for validation of this microRNA panel, showing high sensitivity (96.2%) and specificity (95.1%) for an initial cohort of 200 patients (34). They have now developed a diagnostic tool, Ziwig Endotest®, based on these results. At the time of writing, the multicentre clinical trial is still underway. However, the device is now available in multiple countries, including France and the United Kingdom (35). This diagnostic device highlights how technology and software development, such as next-generation sequencing and artificial intelligence, can further diagnostic capabilities.

Microfluidic devices use small channels, often only tens of micrometres wide, which allow the processing of fluids. The emerging microfluidic technologies have led to the invention of Hera Biotech's MetriDx™, a non-surgical diagnostic test for endometriosis. These analyze proprietary biomarkers in endometrial cells from uterine brush biopsies (36); however, it is in the initial stages of commercialization and is not yet available in the clinics. If successful, MetriDx™ may provide an appropriate screening tool for early diagnosis and staging of the disease.

Overall, conjunctive use of certified biomarkers with imaging and detailed patient information may provide enough diagnostic power to replace laparoscopy as the gold standard. The ambition is to reduce unnecessary surgical procedures, waiting time and pain before diagnosis. While the identification of useful biomarkers has been challenging, there are promising candidates, such as the saliva microRNA panel that could serve as a fingerprint for endometriosis. Most research is moving away from serum analysis towards more local and accessible biofluids, maintaining direct pathology diagnosis. Therefore, research should continue to identify biomarkers in peritoneal fluid, endometrial biopsies and menstrual effluent. However, the successful development of a non-invasive, non-surgical diagnostic device only provides part of the solution. Novel, effective and non-contraceptive treatments are urgently needed to target the underlying disease.

WHAT DOES THE FUTURE HOLD FOR ENDOMETRIOSIS TREATMENTS?

Although laparoscopic surgery and the ablation or excision of identifiable endometriotic lesions improve symptoms and fertility, recovery is often short-lived. Over 60% of women in the UK require repeat operations due to the regrowth of residual endometriosis cells or paradoxically from the formation of surgically induced adhesions (37). Even after surgery, continuous use of oral contraceptives and progestins is recommended for endometriosis-related pain. Since oestrogens play a critical role in disease pathogenesis, these help to shrink lesions. However, they can cause a wide range of side effects, including mood changes, depression, headaches, acne, nausea and thrombosis (38,39). Unravelling the mechanisms and inhibiting lesion growth without the side effects and impact on fertility are major gaps in patient care that researchers aim to address.

ARE THERE ANY PROMISING DRUGS?

Clinical trials of alternative drugs are underway. For example, linzagolix (Yselty®), an oral nonpeptide gonadotropin-releasing hormone (GnRH) antagonist have relatively recently been approved for treatment of uterine fibroids (40). A Phase II/III clinical trial showed that daily doses reduced mean pelvic pain score (non-menstrual pelvic pain and dysmenorrhoea) by over 30% compared with baseline after 12 and 24 weeks in 56.3% to 61.5% of participants (41). This has recently lead to EU approval for broader use of the drug to treat endometriosis symptoms (42). Similarly, Relugolix–estradiol–norethisterone (Ryeqo®) has just been approved by NICE for treating endometriosis-associated pain in the UK as an alternative to injectable GnRH antagonists, that can be taken orally at home (43). However, one serious limitation was a reduction in bone density requiring hormonal add-back therapy limiting the duration of continuous use. Ryeqo, is a combined therapy also replacing the required hormones (43). Elagolix (Orilissa®), the first GnRH oral therapy of this kind is well-tolerated and shows dose-dependent suppression of oestradiol, which allows for individualized dosage and treatment (41). These lessen the hypoestrogenic side effects on bone mineral density and can potentially treat endometriosis without obstructing fertility (42). However, safety data on pregnancy outcomes are currently limited.

NON-HORMONAL, NON-SURGICAL THERAPEUTIC OPTIONS

Non-hormonal drugs that maintain normal ovarian function are needed for the quarter to a third of women with endometriosis who do not respond to first-line therapies and for those trying to conceive (43). Targeting angiogenesis, a hallmark of the disease, using dopamine-receptor 2 agonists is an attractive strategy for treatment. Unlike other antiangiogenic agents, cabergoline reduces prolactin levels, has an acceptable safety profile and does not interfere with menses (44). In a pilot randomized trial, oral cabergoline was well-tolerated and ameliorated pain in women with endometriosis (45). Cabergoline is reported to not increase rates of miscarriage or fetal abnormalities in early pregnancy (46); however, safety data from larger, randomized trials are required.

Another potential breakthrough drug is dichloroacetate, which inhibits the enzyme pyruvate dehydrogenase kinase. In peritoneal cells isolated from women with endometriosis, dichloroacetate targeted metabolic processes, switching from aberrant glycolysis to normal mitochondrial respiration (47). This reversed lactate build-up to control levels and suppressed endometrial cell survival. Oral delivery of dichloroacetate similarly attenuated lactate concentrations and endometriosis lesion size in a mouse model (47), suggesting that targeting this pathway has therapeutic potential. Dichloroacetate has an established safety profile, is licensed for the treatment of rare childhood metabolic disorders and various cancers and seems to be the most promising non-contraceptive drug to recently enter clinical trials.

WHAT ABOUT THE MICROBIOME?

Endometriosis development may also be influenced by the immunologic and biochemical effects of the microbiome (48); consequently, this area of research is increasing in popularity. Lu et al. (2022) investigated bacterial differences in patient vaginal swabs and reported that patients with endometriosis have a decreased population of firmicutes bacteria, particularly *Lactobacillus*, which is favourable to vaginal health by maintaining pH and protecting against pathogenic microorganisms (49,50). Patients also exhibited an increased abundance of actinobacteria (*Atopobium* and *Gardnerella*), which is harmful, compared to controls. This change in bacterial composition (dysbiosis) is similar to that encountered in bacterial vaginosis. In contrast, a different form of dysbiosis was discovered, whereby patients with confirmed stage III and IV endometriosis, as classified by the American Fertility Society (51), lacked *Atopobium* in their vaginal microbiome (48). Muraoka et al. (2023) found that *Fusobacterium* was elevated in 64% of patients with endometriosis compared to a control group in which merely 7% had similarly high levels (52). Interestingly, they also found a higher frequency of *Fusobacterium* inside the endometriotic lesions and endometrial tissues of patients with endometriosis compared to controls, suggesting that this bacterial species plays a pathogenic role. However, the relationship between the microbiome and development of endometriosis remains unclear.

In a mouse model created through peritoneal injection of donor mouse endometrial tissue, antibiotic treatment against *Fusobacterium* reduced endometriotic lesion weight (52). Lu et al. (2022) used a similar in vivo model to either transplant vaginal microbiota from healthy mice to those induced with endometriosis or administer antibiotics as a treatment (49). Both methods attenuated lesion size and progression. This highlights a potential new therapeutic avenue for endometriosis with the use of antibiotics or microbiota transplantations within the vaginal tract, similar to that used for colitis (53).

The microbiomes in the peritoneum, gut and uterus are also being investigated (54). Even so, research into differences in the microbiome remains elusive as it is relatively new. The variance in microbiome dysbiosis may be due to differences in diet, ethnicity, type or severity of endometriosis, menstrual cycle phase, or simply a limited number of research participants. Therefore, it is important to recruit diverse cohorts so that overall trends can be fully investigated. The potential development of alternative antibiotic or microbiota treatments is exciting as more insights are uncovered. Once the microbiome correlations are substantially characterized, the challenge will be to devise a delivery system consisting of either microbiota cocktails or specific antibiotics in order to determine their clinical relevance in alleviating endometriosis in patients.

NANOMEDICINES: ARE THEY THE BEST TYPE OF TREATMENT?

Alternative drug delivery methods, such as nanoparticles, are needed to enhance efficacy, reduce adverse effects and improve compliance with pharmacotherapy approaches to treating endometriosis (55,56). Since endometriosis is an angiogenic disease, requiring increased vasculature for the implantation, growth and survival of endometriotic lesions, inhibition by angiostatic agents is beneficial (56–58). Increased vascularization is associated with enhanced permeability and retention of nanoparticles, making endometriotic lesions an ideal target for nanomedicines (56).

Nanoparticles have been explored for use in a wide range of therapies (55). Nanotechnologies composed of bioconjugates have demonstrated an ability to deliver anti-angiogenic, antioxidant, immunomodulating and anti-inflammatory molecules to endometriotic lesions in mouse models (55).

Boroumand et al. (2020) investigated the use of a local curcumin treatment, delivered in polymer nanofibers to the peritoneum of an endometriosis mouse model (59). Curcumin, derived from turmeric plants, abrogates endometriotic lesion growth by inhibiting oestradiol production (60). The nanofibers promoted sustained release of curcumin over 30 days and promoted histological changes, including reducing the number of endometrial glands and stroma. Sustained drug release was also successful in mouse and rat endometriosis models using glycolipid-like polymer micelles delivery systems (61).

OUR RESEARCH AND THE NEXT STEPS

The pelvic peritoneal space, which functions to protect and support abdominal organs, is of considerable interest to our research group at the University of Manchester. It is immunologically dynamic and links the reproductive and endocrine systems, contributing to pathogenesis and progression of disease. Factors that predispose women to endometriosis, adenomyosis and adhesion formation are especially important, including differences in immunosurveillance, haemostasis, inflammation, cell proliferation and tissue remodelling. In the laboratory we use a combination of patient biopsies, in vitro cell models and mouse models of endometriosis and endometriosis recurrence to study the uterine and lesion environments as well as the effects of drugs. These help us to understand the drivers, find potential therapeutic targets and develop solutions for this unmet clinical need.

Importantly, we also investigate non-hormonal therapies and new ways to target endometriosis sites to reduce systemic side effects (58,62,63). This would be revolutionary for patients prioritizing fertility. Formulations are

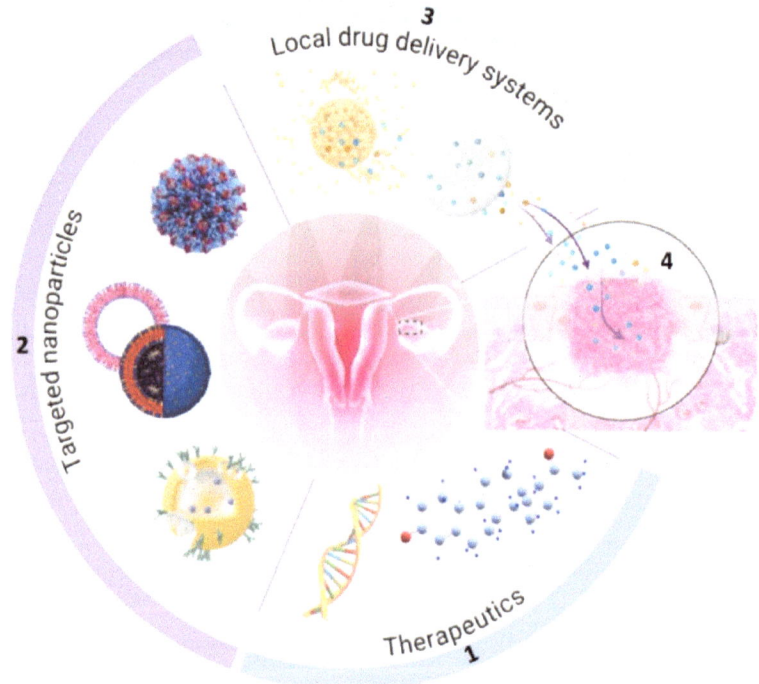

FIGURE 19.1 The future of precision medicine for endometriosis is moving towards (1) hormone and non-hormonal medicines, as well as immuno- and gene therapies based on patient diagnosis, symptoms and response to treatment. The challenge is to overcome their inherent instability, insolubility and toxicity. (2) One way is to deliver these medicines in nanoparticle carriers like micelles, liposomes, polymeric nanospheres and dendrimers, designed to target diseased cells. (3) Another is to use local drug delivery systems, such as nanoemulsions or hydrogels, which are administered to (4) endometriosis sites and effectively transport active ingredients and gene fragments by passive or active diffusion. Controlled delivery of these tailored treatments should enhance therapeutic performance whilst minimizing harm to healthy tissues.

becoming more sophisticated, whether they be lipid-based carriers, such as liposomes and micelles, decorated nanoparticles or hydrogel biomaterials for controlled localized delivery of drugs, immunotherapies or gene therapies (Figure 19.1). These could be used to overcome the limitations of traditional pharmaceutical compounds and medical devices, transforming how endometriosis is treated for millions of women.

The next frontier in endometriosis research is personalized medicine. Treatments are moving from a one-size-fits-all standard-of-care to a more targeted approach based on unique patient characteristics. By working with GPs, pharmacists and clinical collaborators, researchers are capturing information about patients' personal and clinical history, correlating them with genomic profiles and responsiveness to drugs. In this age of digital technology and artificial intelligence, the ultimate aim is to develop a medical model for defined groups of individuals. Customizing more effective prevention, diagnostic and treatment strategies within clinical practice would be ground-breaking.

CONCLUSION

Whilst current hormonal therapies can help to alleviate symptoms, they fail to address issues with fertility. This is compounded by high rates of post-surgical recurrence, leaving many patients with debilitating symptoms that impact their physical and mental wellbeing. One reason for slow progress until now has been the marginalization and stigma about endometriosis as well as chronic underfunding in this area. The recent shift in the prominence of women's reproductive health, however, is fuelling new research.

Throughout this chapter, we have introduced some innovations in endometriosis research and potential diagnostic and treatment options that may be on the horizon. Non-hormonal therapies and new drug delivery strategies are exciting avenues that could provide safe and effective treatments without undesirable side effects.

Endometriosis is a complex disorder and research can only succeed through collaboration. At the University of Manchester, we are extremely fortunate to have strong ties with the Northern Care Alliance Endometriosis Centre, headed by Miss Gaity Ahmad, and Professor Emma Crosbie and her Obstetrics and Gynaecology team at St Mary's Hospital, Manchester. Not only do they actively recruit participants and collect research specimens, they also provide invaluable insights into the feasibility of medical devices in the clinical setting. We have been completely overwhelmed by the kindness, strength and eager participation of patients who enrol in these research studies and clinical trials, even when they often do not personally benefit from the outcome. Given the huge interest and generosity of the patients we have encountered, and passion of researchers, clinicians, the public and policymakers, new diagnosis and treatments cannot be too far away.

KEY POINT SUMMARY

- Research must be translated into practice to reduce delays in diagnosis, improve patient quality of life and reduce the economic burden of endometriosis.
- Promising panels of biomarkers are being analyzed in saliva and menstrual fluid but may prove most useful in combination with imaging techniques.
- Potential treatments for endometriosis are broad and cover many different avenues, including new and repurposed drugs as well as targeted delivery methods.
- Collaboration between health care professionals and researchers is paramount to effectively shape endometriosis research.

REFERENCES

1. Zondervan KT, Becker CM, Missmer SA. Endometriosis. *N Engl J Med* 2020 Mar 26;382(13):1244–56. Mirin AA. Gender disparity in the funding of diseases by the U.S. National Institutes of Health. *J Womens Health (Larchmt)* 2021 Jul;30(7):956–63.
2. Smith, K. Women's health research lacks funding—these charts show how. *Nature* 2023;617:28–9.
3. Estimates of Funding for Various Research, Condition, and Disease Categories (RCDC). https://report.nih.gov/funding/categorical-spending#/2022
4. UK Health Research Analysis 2018; UK Clinical Research Collaboration, 2020. https://hrcsonline.net/reports/analysis-reports/uk-health-research-analysis-2018/
5. Zondervan KT, Becker CM, Missmer SA. Endometriosis. *N Engl J Med* 2020 Mar 26;382(13):1244–56.
6. All Party Parliamentary Group (APPG). Endometriosis in the UK: Time for Change. APPG on Endometriosis Inquiry Report. 2020. https://www.endometriosis-uk.org/appg-release-new-report-endometriosis#_ftn1
7. Simoens S, Dunselman G, Dirksen C, et al. The burden of endometriosis: Costs and quality of life of women with endometriosis and treated in referral centres. *Hum Reprod* 2012;27(5):1292–9.
8. Nisenblat V, Bossuyt PM, Farquhar C, et al. Imaging modalities for the non-invasive diagnosis of endometriosis. *Cochrane Database Syst Rev* 2016;(2).
9. Kiesel L, Sourouni M. Diagnosis of endometriosis in the 21st century. *Climacteric* 2019 Jun;22(3):296–302.
10. Chapron C, Marcellin L, Borghese B et al. Rethinking mechanisms, diagnosis and management of endometriosis. *Nat Rev Endocrinol* 2019; 15(11):666–82.

11. Oldan J. Evaluation of endometriosis with 18F-fluoroestradiol PET/MRI, Clinicaltrials.gov. 2023. https://clinicaltrials.gov/study/NCT04382911?con d=Endometriosis&rank=1&limit=10&aggFilters=results%3Awith%2Cstat us%3Acom&tab=history&a=14#more-information-card (accessed 26 Oct 2023).

12. Leonardi M. Combining ultrasound and biomarkers to diagnose superficial endometriosis (SPGENDO). *ClinicalTrials.gov.* 2023. https://clinicaltrials. gov/study/NCT05523284?cond=Endometriosis&term=Combining+ ultrasound+and+biomarkers+to+diagnose+superficial+endometriosis+ &rank=1#publications (accessed 18 Oct 2023).

13. Ianieri MM, Della Corte L, Campolo F, et al. Indocyanine green in the surgical management of endometriosis: A systematic review. *Acta Obstet Gynecol Scand* 2021;100(2):189–99.

14. Cosentino F, Vizzielli G, Turco LC, et al. Near-infrared imaging with indocyanine green for detection of endometriosis lesions (Gre-Endo Trial): A pilot study. *J Minim Invasive Gynecol* 2018;25:1249–54.

15. Malutan AM, Drugan T, Costin N, et al. Pro-inflammatory cytokines for evaluation of inflammatory status in endometriosis. *Eur J Immunol* 2015;40(1):96–102.

16. Sharpe-Timms KL, Nabli H, Zimmer RL, et al. Inflammatory cytokines differentially up-regulate human endometrial haptoglobin production in women with endometriosis. *Hum Reprod* 2010 May 1;25(5):1241–50.

17. Kokot I, Piwowar A, Jędryka M et al. Diagnostic significance of selected serum inflammatory markers in women with advanced endometriosis. *Int J Mol Sci*, 2021;22(5):2295.

18. Cheng YM, Wang ST, Chou CY. Serum CA-125 in preoperative patients at high risk for endometriosis. *Obstet Gynecol* 2002;99(3):375–80.

19. Karimi-Zarchi M, Dehshiri-Zadeh N, Sekhavat L, et al. Correlation of CA-125 serum level and clinico-pathological characteristic of patients with endometriosis. *Int J Reprod Biomed*, 2016;14(11):713.

20. Charkhchi P, Cybulski C, Gronwald J, et al. CA125 and ovarian cancer: A comprehensive review. *Cancers* 2020;12(12):3730.

21. Jiang T, Huang L, Zhang S. Preoperative serum CA125: A useful marker for surgical management of endometrial cancer. *BMC Cancer* 2015;15(1):1–8.

22. Babacan A, Kizilaslan C, Gun I, et al. CA 125 and other tumor markers in uterine leiomyomas and their association with lesion characteristics. *Int J Clin Exp Med* 2014;7(4):1078.

23. King GL. The role of inflammatory cytokines in diabetes and its complications. *J Periodontol* 2008;79:1527–34.

24. Pradhan AD, Manson JE, Rifai N, et al. C-reactive protein, interleukin 6, and risk of developing type 2 diabetes mellitus. *JAMA* 2001;286(3):327–34.

25. Borthakur A, Prabhu YD, Gopalakrishnan AV. Role of IL-6 signalling in polycystic ovarian syndrome associated inflammation. *J Reprod Immunol* 2020;141:103155.

26. Rostamtabar M, Esmaeilzadeh S, Tourani M, et al. Pathophysiological roles of chronic low-grade inflammation mediators in polycystic ovary syndrome. *J Cell Physiol* 2021;236(2):824–38.

27. Choghakhori R, Abbasnezhad A, Hasanvand A, et al. Inflammatory cytokines and oxidative stress biomarkers in irritable bowel syndrome: Association with digestive symptoms and quality of life. *Cytokine* 2017;93:34–43.

28. Eisenberg VH, Decter DH, Chodick G, et al. Burden of endometriosis: Infertility, comorbidities, and healthcare resource utilization. *J Clin Med* 2022;11(4):1133.

29. Ahn SH, Singh V, Tayade C. Biomarkers in endometriosis: Challenges and opportunities. *Fertil Steril* 2017;107(3):523–32.
30. Hewitt SC, Dickson MJ, Edwards N, et al. From cup to dish: How to make and use endometrial organoid and stromal cultures derived from menstrual fluid. *Front Endocrinol* 2023;14.
31. Shih AJ, Adelson RP, Vashistha H, et al. Single-cell analysis of menstrual endometrial tissues defines phenotypes associated with endometriosis. *BMC Medicine* 2022;20(1):1–16.
32. Gregersen PK. *Research OutSmarts Endometriosis II Study (ROSE2), CTG Labs—NCBI*. https://clinicaltrials.gov/study/NCT05601596 (accessed 24 Oct 2023).
33. Bendifallah S, Suisse S, Puchar A, et al. Salivary microRNA signature for diagnosis of endometriosis. *J Clin Med* 2022;11(3):612.
34. Bendifallah S, Dabi Y, Suisse S, et al. Validation of a salivary miRNA signature of endometriosis—Interim data. *NEJM Evidence* 2023;2(7):EVIDoa2200282.
35. French health authorities fast-track reimbursement for Ziwig saliva endometriosis test (2025) *Femtech Insider*. Available at: https://femtechinsider. com/french-health-authorities-fast-track-reimbursement-for-ziwig-saliva-endometriosis-test/?utm_source=chatgpt.com (Accessed: 06 March 2025).
36. Robinson JA. Proof of concept study to eval MetriDx lab-developed test to identify endometriosis-specific bio markers. *ClinicalTrials.gov.* https:// clinicaltrials.gov/study/NCT05698212?cond=Endometriosis&intr=Diagno stic+Test&rank=1 (accessed 18 Oct 2023).
37. Li XY, Chao XP, Leng JH, Zhang W, et al. Risk factors for postoperative recurrence of ovarian endometriosis: Long-term follow-up of 358 women. *J Ovarian Res*, 2019;12:1–10.
38. Skovlund CW, Mørch LS, Kessing LV, et al. Association of hormonal contraception with depression. *JAMA Psychiatry* 2016;73(11):1154–62.
39. Skovlund CW, Mørch LS, Kessing LV, et al. Association of hormonal contraception with suicide attempts and suicides. *Am J Psychiatry* 2018;175(4):336–42.
40. National Institute for Health and Care Excellence. Linzagolix for treating moderate to severe symptoms of uterine fibroids. 14 Aug 2024. https:// www.nice.org.uk/guidance/ta996
41. Donnez J, Taylor HS, Taylor RN, et al. Treatment of endometriosis-associated pain with linzagolix, an oral gonadotropin-releasing hormone–antagonist: A randomized clinical trial. *Fertil Steril* 2020;114(1):44–55.
42. European Medicines Agency. YSELTY EU SmPC. Available at: https://www. ema.europa.eu/en/medicines/human/EPAR/yselty Last accessed: March 2025
43. National Institute for Health and Care Excellence. First daily pill for endometriosis approved for NHS use. 13 March 2025. https://www.nice.org.uk/ news/articles/first-daily-pill-for-endometriosis-approved-for-nhs-use Last accesses: March 2025.
44. Yan H, Shi J, Li X, et al. Oral gonadotropin-releasing hormone antagonists for treating endometriosis-associated pain: A systematic review and network meta-analysis. *Fertil Steril* 2022 Dec;118(6):1102–16.
45. Leyland N, Estes SJ, Lessey BA, et al. A clinician's guide to the treatment of endometriosis with elagolix. *J Womens Health (Larchmt)* 2021 Apr;30(4):569–78.
46. Becker CM, Gattrell WT, Gude K, et al. Reevaluating response and failure of medical treatment of endometriosis: A systematic review. *Fertil Steril* 2017;108:125–36.

47. Yarmolinskaya M, Suslova E, Tkachenko N, et al. Dopamine agonists as genital endometriosis target therapy. *Gynecol Endocrinol* 2020;36(sup1):7–11.

48. DiVasta AD, Stamoulis C, Gallagher JS, et al. Nonhormonal therapy for endometriosis: A randomized, placebo-controlled, pilot study of cabergoline versus norethindrone acetate. *F S Rep* 2021 Jul 24;2(4):454–61.

49. Colao A, Abs R, Bárcena DG, et al. Pregnancy outcomes following cabergoline treatment: Extended results from a 12-year observational study. *Clin Endocrinol (Oxf)* 2008 Jan;68(1):66–71. doi:10.1111/j.1365-2265.2007.03000.x. Epub 2007 Aug 29. pmid:17760883.

50. Horne AW, Ahmad SF, Carter R, et al. Repurposing dichloroacetate for the treatment of women with endometriosis. *Proc Natl Acad Sci U S A* 2019 Dec 17;116(51):25389–91.

51. Ata B, Yildiz S, Turkgeldi E, et al. The endobiota study: Comparison of vaginal, cervical and gut microbiota between women with stage 3/4 endometriosis and healthy controls. *Sci Rep* 2019;9(1):2204.

52. Lu F, Wei J, Zhong Y, et al. Antibiotic therapy and vaginal microbiota transplantation reduce endometriosis disease progression in female mice via NF-κB signaling pathway. *Front Med* 2022;9:831115.

53. Wei W, Zhang X, Tang H, et al. Microbiota composition and distribution along the female reproductive tract of women with endometriosis. *Ann Clin Microbiol Antimicrob* 2020;19:1–8.

54. Canis M, Donnez JG, Guzick DS, et al. Revised American Society for Reproductive Medicine classification of endometriosis: 1996. *Fertil Steril* 1997;67(5):817–21.

55. Muraoka A, Suzuki M, Hamaguchi T, et al. Fusobacterium infection facilitates the development of endometriosis through the phenotypic transition of endometrial fibroblasts. *Sci Transl Med* 2023;15(700):eadd1531.

56. Borody TJ, Khoruts A. Fecal microbiota transplantation and emerging applications. *Nat Rev Gastroenterol Hepatol* 2012;9(2):88–96.

57. Yuan W, Wu Y, Chai X, et al. The colonized microbiota composition in the peritoneal fluid in women with endometriosis. *Arch Gynecol Obstet* 2022:1–8.

58. Garzon S, Laganà AS, Barra F, et al. Novel drug delivery methods for improving efficacy of endometriosis treatments. *Expert Opin Drug Deliv* 2021 18(3):355–67.

59. Moses AS, Demessie AA, Taratula O, et al. Nanomedicines for endometriosis: Lessons learned from cancer research. *Small* 2021;17(7):2004975.

60. Nap AW, Griffioen AW, Dunselman GA, et al. Antiangiogenesis therapy for endometriosis. *J Clin Endocrinol Metab* 2004;89(3):1089–95.

61. Santorelli S, Fischer DP, Harte MK, et al. In vivo effects of AZD4547, a novel fibroblast growth factor receptor inhibitor, in a mouse model of endometriosis. *Pharmacol Res Perspect* 2021;9(2):e00759.

62. Boroumand S, Hosseini S, Pashandi Z, et al. Curcumin-loaded nanofibers for targeting endometriosis in the peritoneum of a mouse model. *J Mater Sci: Mater Med* 2020;31:1–9.

63. Zhang Y, Cao H, Yu Z, et al. Curcumin inhibits endometriosis endometrial cells by reducing estradiol production. *Iran J Reprod Med* 2013;11(5):415.

64. Yuan M, Ding S, Meng T, et al. Effect of A-317491 delivered by glycolipid-like polymer micelles on endometriosis pain. *Int J Nanomed* 2017:8171–83.

65. Kitson SJ, Rosser M, Fischer DP, et al. Targeting endometrial cancer stem cell activity with metformin is inhibited by patient-derived adipocyte-secreted factors. *Cancers* 2019;11(5):653.

66. Fischer DP, Griffiths AL, Lui S, et al. Distribution and function of prosta-glandin E2 receptors in mouse uterus: Translational value for human repro-duction. *J Pharmacol Exp Ther* 2020 Jun;373(3):381–90.

FURTHER READING

UK Health Research Analysis 2018. UK Clinical Research Collaboration. 2020. https://hrcsonline.net/reports/analysis-reports/uk-health-research-analy-sis-2018/

CHAPTER 20

Clinical Trials in the UK

....

Clinical trials enable researchers to investigate new ways of treating and managing endometriosis and compare two or more types of treatment to see what works best. They are run by doctors and researchers, in one or more hospitals across the UK.

Each trial has a patient information sheet for patients taking part in the trial to understand and discuss with the doctor and research nurses about the trial.

Endometriosis trials are led by the Centre for Excellence in Pelvic Pain and Endometriosis Care and Treatment (EXPECT), which draws on expertise from the Centre for Inflammatory Research (CIR) and the Centre for Reproductive Health (CRH). The EXPECT project is co-directed by Professor Andrew Horne and Professor Philippa Saunders from the Centre for Inflammatory Research (1).

VARIOUS CLINICAL TRIALS

Recent research has brought new hopes for those suffering from this debilitating condition. From non-hormonal treatments to immunotherapy, researchers are working tirelessly to improve diagnosis and treatment options.

As awareness and funding for endometriosis research and trials continue to grow, we are hopeful to see even more innovative solutions to manage this complex and multifaceted condition.

Advances in organoids and the role of the microbiome and diet are leading to new diagnostics and treatments for endometriosis, motivating a precision health approach to this long-neglected disease (2).

DOI: 10.1201/9781032684819-26

1. *ESPriT2: Effectiveness of Laparoscopic Removal of Superficial Peritoneal Endometriosis for the Management of Chronic Pelvic Pain*

   This trial is run by the University of Edinburgh. **ESPriT2** is a randomized controlled trial to determine whether laparoscopic removal of isolated superficial peritoneal endometriosis (SPE) by excision or ablation is of benefit for the management of chronic pelvic pain.

   Isolated superficial peritoneal endometriosis means that no deep endometriosis has been found on organs such as the bowel, only endometriosis on the peritoneal lining of the pelvic cavity.

   The study will compare patients with superficial peritoneal endometriosis who have had endometriosis surgically removed via laparoscopy with patients who have had only a diagnostic laparoscopy (i.e., no removal surgery took place). Participants will be randomly assigned to having diagnostic laparoscopy only or laparoscopy and removal and will not know which procedure they had.

   Researchers will also be able to compare patient outcomes for different methods of laparoscopic removal of endometriosis, namely ablation and excision (3).

2. *REGAL: Recurrence of Endometriosis: Clinical and Cost-Effectiveness of Gonadotropin-Releasing Hormone Analogues with Add-Back HRT versus Repeat Laparoscopic Surgery*

   REGAL is a clinical trial considering how best to treat those who have already had surgery for endometriosis but then later experience recurrence of endometriosis pain. The trial will compare further surgery versus hormonal treatment and is run by the University of Aberdeen.

   This randomized controlled trial will compare long-term GnRH analogues (hormones which temporarily stop the ovaries producing oestrogen, "medical menopause") with added HRT to keyhole surgery in women who experience recurrence of endometriosis pain after surgery but who wish to preserve their fertility.

   Eligibility criteria to take part includes having recurrent pain following laparoscopic treatment for endometriosis and being 21–49 years old (3–5).

   Further information including study sites and how to take part can be found on the REGAL website: https://w3.abdn.ac.uk/hsru/REGAL.

3. *DIAMOND: Deep-Infiltrating Endometriosis: Management by Medical Treatment versus Early Surgery*

This trial compares the effectiveness of medical management (hormones) and surgery for deep endometriosis and is run by the University of Aberdeen and the University of Birmingham.

It is a randomized controlled trial (RCT) comparing management of deep-infiltrating endometriosis by medical treatment versus early surgery. The study will compare early planned laparoscopic surgery (with or without medical treatment alongside or afterwards) versus medical management alone in women with deep-infiltrating endometriosis.

Eligibility criteria include those aged 18–49 seeking treatment for pain with confirmed deep endometriosis and suitable for either surgical or medical management (6). Further information including study sites and how to take part can be found on the DIAMOND website.

4. *Dichloroacetate*: Researchers at the University of Edinburgh have announced results of a study suggesting the painful symptoms of endometriosis could be treated with the drug dichloroacetate (7).

Lead Researcher, Professor Andrew Horne, MRC Centre for Reproductive Health at University of Edinburgh, said:

> *Endometriosis can be a life-changing condition for so many women. Now that we understand better the metabolism of the cells in women that have endometriosis, we can work to develop a non-hormonal treatment. Through a clinical trial with dichloroacetate we should be able to see if the conditions we observed in the lab are replicated in women with endometriosis.*

The researchers believe these new findings could help ease endometriosis in women who cannot or do not wish to take hormonal treatments or prevent recurrence of the disease after surgery. The team are conducting an early phase clinical trial to see if they can confirm their findings. Clinical trials are medical research studies involving people, designed to find out if a treatment or procedure is safe, has side effects, works better than the currently used treatment and affects quality of life; clinical trials are essential in the development of potential treatments.

The research team have found that cells from the pelvic wall of women with endometriosis have a different metabolism compared to women without the disease. The cells produced higher amounts of lactate—a potentially harmful waste product—which is like the behaviour of cancer cells.

In laboratory tests, treating cells of women with endometriosis with dichloroacetate was found to lower the production of lactate and return the cells to normal metabolic function.

Further testing in mice with endometriosis found that dichloroacetate, after 7 days of treatment, caused a marked reduction in pelvic lactate concentrations and the size of the lesions. Dichloroacetate is a drug that is used to treat rare metabolic disorders in children and has previously been investigated as a cancer treatment. Following these laboratory studies, 30 women with endometriosis were treated with dichloroacetate (a trial called EPiC1). The women in this small trial reported that they had less painful symptoms and required fewer painkillers when they were taking dichloroacetate.

Some of the women described the treatment as "life changing," but some women had mild side effects, like heartburn/nausea or tingling in their fingers.

The researchers are now planning to test dichloroacetate in a bigger trial (called EPiC2) of 100 women from two Scottish hospitals with endometriosis and compare it to a placebo ("dummy" tablets). The aim of the EPiC2 trial is to learn what dose of dichloroacetate has the most impact on painful endometriosis symptoms and has the fewest side effects. The data from EPiC2 will also help plan a future larger UK-wide trial to truly determine whether dichloroacetate can reduce endometriosis-associated pain, improve quality of life and provide value for money.

Assuming that EPiC2 is completed in 2025, this larger trial could provide definitive results by 2030.

The aim is if dichloroacetate is shown to be truly effective, it will be rapidly incorporated into national and international recommendations for the treatment of women with endometriosis. EPiC2 will be analyzed to find out what dose of dichloroacetate has the most impact on painful endometriosis symptoms and has the fewest side effects.

5. *Endo-Tect: Urine test*: A new urine test developed by the University of Hull has identified proteins that are increased in the urine of women suffering from endometriosis. It is not available to the public yet, but this test called EndoTect will take seconds to indicate whether endometriosis is the cause of the symptoms a patient is experiencing.

This test can also indicate whether the patient has superficial or deep endometriosis and monitor the effectiveness of treatment. Although the test is still being developed, it is hoped it will be available to the public in 2–3 years, hopefully through the NHS (8).

6. *Endometriosis drug trial*: The Gynaecology and Research and Development team at Norfolk and Norwich University Hospital (NNUH) are playing a key role in leading a Phase II research study, which will evaluate an antibody designed to reduce inflammation and endometriosis symptoms (9).

The first patient has taken part in the AMY109EU (ACERS; Assessing a new treatment Concept for EndometRioSis) study which is trialling the safety and effectiveness of an antibody called AMY109, which has been developed by scientists from Chugai Pharmaceutical Co Ltd.

The drug blocks a protein (interleukin-8) that promotes the body's inflammatory response to endometriosis.

The way that AMY109 works in reducing inflammation and potentially the destructive scarring of endometriosis could mean, in the long-term, that some women may avoid surgery for this debilitating disease.

Other hospitals in the UK are also taking part in this study, and potential participants may be able to take part in the randomized study if they:

○ Are female aged 18–49
○ Have endometriosis previously diagnosed by laparoscopy (incision made in the abdomen and a thin tube with a camera [laparoscope] inserted to look for lesions, adhesions and endometrioma [cyst/s])
○ Willing to have laparoscopic surgery after study treatment

Paul Simpson, Consultant Gynaecologist, who is the Principal Investigator at NNUH, added:

> *Everything so far in the treatment of endometriosis has suppressed the disease symptoms, but this new drug addresses inflammation and potentially reverse the effects of endometriosis without the need for surgery. It is different to every other available treatment for endometriosis because it could be disease modifying. Antibody based treatments are widely used in health care for treating some cancers and chronic inflammatory conditions such as, rheumatoid arthritis and inflammatory bowel disease.*

Phase I trials of the antibody have involved healthy volunteers and patients in Japan and Taiwan.

Whilst this potential new drug is at an early stage in its development, the researchers hope it will not only reduce inflammation caused by endometriosis but may potentially reduce scarring that has already occurred. With the added benefit of being non-hormonal, it could be also available to those for whom contraceptives are not suitable.

KEY POINT SUMMARY

- Research is needed towards finding the cause of endometriosis so that better treatment and management can be provided and perhaps a cure.
- Clinical trials enable researchers to investigate new ways of treating and managing endometriosis; and comparing two or more types of treatment to see what works best. They are run by doctors and researchers, in one or more hospitals across the UK.
- Research into effective endometriosis treatment is hampered by widespread variations in outcome reporting and short durations of investigation.
- Collaboration is needed between researchers and clinicians to conduct large-scale well-designed trials of adequate duration to further guide clinical decision-making.
- Without significant investment in research, patients with endometriosis will continue to face delays in accessing the right treatment at the right time.

REFERENCES

1. Watson, Clare. Surge in endometriosis research after decades of underfunding could herald new era for women's health. *Nat Med* 2024 Feb;30(2):315–18. doi:10.1038/s41591-024-02795-0. pubmed.ncbi.nlm.nih.gov/3832121
2. Donhong Y, Cao H, Wang X. Advances and applications of organoids: A review. *Sheng Wu Gong Cheng Xue Bao*. 2021 Nov 25;37(11): 3961–74. doi:10.13345/j.cjb.200764
3. www.ed.ac.uk/centre-reproductive-health/espirit2 ESPriT2/The University of Edinburgh.
4. W3.abdn.ac.uk/hsru/REGAL.
5. REGAL website. https://w3.abdn.ac.uk/hsru/REGAL/Public/Public/index.cshtml
6. DIAMOND website. https://w3.abdn.ac.uk/hsru/DIAMOND. DIAMOND-University of Aberdeen.
7. www.ed.ac.uk/research/epic2-clinical-Trial EPiC2 Clinical Trial/The University of Edinburgh.
8. Patient.info/news-and-features/what-we-know/New Endometriosis test could reduce diagnosis times by years.
9. www.femtechworld.co.uk/news/uk-hospital-launches: UK hospital launches 'world-first' endometriosis study.

CHAPTER 21

Current Challenges and Future Prospects

....

In many countries, the general public and most frontline health care providers are not aware that distressing and life-altering pelvic pain is not normal, leading to a normalization and stigmatization of symptoms and significant diagnostic delay (1,2).

Patients who could benefit from medical symptomatic management are not always provided with treatments due to limited awareness of endometriosis among primary health care providers. Due to diagnostic delays, prompt access to available treatment methods, including nonsteroidal analgesics (painkillers), oral contraceptives and progestin-based contraceptives is often not achieved. The impact on quality of life can be huge, and in one survey, 95% said endometriosis had impacted their lives negatively or very negatively (3)

Due to the limited capacity of health systems in many countries, access to specialized surgery for those who need it is suboptimal. In addition, and especially in low and middle-income countries, there is a lack of multidisciplinary teams with the wide range of skills and equipment needed for the early diagnosis and effective treatment of endometriosis.

Despite the prevalence and the severity of the condition, there remain many challenges in endometriosis care, with delayed diagnosis, a lack of patient-friendly diagnostics and a need for more targeted treatments.

DOI: 10.1201/9781032684819-27

WHAT ARE THE CHALLENGES AND WHY IS IT MISSED?

Clinical Diagnosis

Clinical diagnosis is difficult, partly because of non-specific symptoms, and may be attributed to other conditions; for example, endometriosis may mimic or cause irritable bowel syndrome (4).

Symptoms may be misdiagnosed as functional or psychosomatic (3) or dismissed. Women constantly report difficulties in convincing doctors about the severity of symptoms (3).

Despite increased public awareness and clinical education, early recognition of endometriosis remains uncommon, possibly because of gaps in evidence about the clinical relevance of mild disease at laparoscopy, poor correlation between symptoms and extent of disease, the need for histological confirmation, limited laparoscopy access and/or laparoscopy cost (5).

Across the UK, there is some excellent treatment provided, including prompt diagnosis and follow-up, but this is not the case for everyone.

Retrospective data analysis in the UK showed that one-third of patients had consulted their GP six times or more before referral, with 39% having two or more gynaecological referrals before receiving a definitive diagnosis (6).

Diagnostic delay is even more common in adolescents (7), possibly because of the unfounded belief that endometriosis takes time to cause symptoms after menarche (8).

Of those studied, 89% felt isolated due to endometriosis and 58% would have liked fertility support and treatment but were not offered (endometriosis doubles the infertility risk) (9).

Cultural Barriers

Cultural barriers to discussing menstruation and sexual symptoms still exist and may cause reluctance or difficulty in reporting them (3). The lack of reliable non-invasive tests likely also contributes to delays (10,11). This is intensified by the variation and methodological quality of endometriosis guidelines, which suggest different diagnostic criteria (12).

Gaps in Research

This is the real issue. A lack of medical research means that we still do not know what the causes of endometriosis are and what is the good treatment. The US National Institutes of Health (NIH) had a budget just shy of $42 billion in 2020 and only $13 million of that went to endometriosis research. The NIH invests most of its nearly $48 billion budget in medical research for the American people. Nearly 83% of NIH's funding is awarded for extramural research, largely through almost 50,000 competitive grants to more than 300,000 researchers at more than 2,500 universities, medical schools and other research institutions in every state. In addition, approximately 11% of the NIH's budget supports projects conducted by nearly 6,000 scientists in its own laboratories, most of which are on the NIH campus in Bethesda, Maryland. The remaining 6% covers research support, administrative and facility construction, maintenance or operational costs. This puts it below funding into teenage pregnancy and teenage sexual activity (13). This is part of a broader problem of a lack of funding for women's health issues generally, with less than 2.5% of funding in the UK going into the area.

Lack of Treatments

There is no cure for endometriosis, and it can be difficult to treat. The mainstay of treatment currently is pain medications, oral contraceptives or surgery.

Pain medications are useful but fail to address the underlying problem, and there is some conflicting evidence for oral contraceptive use.

There are several medications currently in animal studies and phase I–II clinical trials (6). Hopefully, these can offer future solutions.

As laid out by a recent APPG report (3) about endometriosis, there is a considerable need for novel non-hormonal targeted therapies that would relieve pain, allow the menstrual cycle to continue and, ideally, allow for pregnancy during treatment and prevent recurrence by targeting specific disease-associated pathways.

WHY DOES IT MATTER?

In many countries, the public and most frontline health care providers are not aware that distressing and life-altering pelvic pain is not normal, leading to a normalization and stigmatization of symptoms and significant diagnostic delay. Patients who could benefit from medical symptomatic management are not always provided with treatments due to limited awareness of this condition among primary health care providers (GPs).

It is unknown whether earlier treatment affects the course of endometriosis or reduces the incidence of chronic pain, but delay in diagnosis of endometriosis can cause considerable suffering, distress, impaired quality of life, economic hardship, reduced productivity and reduced workforce participation (14,15).

In the UK, work absenteeism and health care costs related to endometriosis cause economic losses of around £8.2 billion a year (direct treatment costs are comparable to those for type 2 diabetes and rheumatoid arthritis) (16).

Due to diagnostic delays, prompt access to available treatment including nonsteroidal analgesics, oral contraceptives and progestin-based contraceptives is often not achieved. Earlier diagnosis and prompt treatment might reduce psychosocial and economic burdens (17).

Due to the limited capacity of the health system (shortage of specialized surgeons in endometriosis), access to specialized surgery for those who need it is suboptimal.

Although primary health care professionals should play a role in screening and basic management of endometriosis, tools to screen and accurately predict patients and populations who are most likely to have the disease are lacking. In addition, many knowledge gaps exist, and there is need for non-invasive diagnostic methods as well as medical treatments that do not prevent pregnancy.

According to retrospective population-linked data, delayed diagnosis was associated with a reduced chance of pregnancy by 33% in those who required assisted reproductive technology (17).

HOPE FOR THE FUTURE

While still a stigmatized and little-known condition, endometriosis is beginning to garner more attention because of the report published by APPG and WHO mentioning the priorities related to endometriosis.

Report by the All-Party Parliamentary Group (APPG)

The APPG will not rest until tangible improvements are delivered to all those who suffer from this condition. Action is needed now, to ensure the next generation with endometriosis are not robbed of the future they deserve.

An Inquiry by the All-Party Parliamentary Group UK (APPG) on Endometriosis has highlighted the devastating impact endometriosis can have on all aspects of a person's life and is urging Ministers to take bold action to ensure those with endometriosis have access to the right care at the right time.

The inquiry surveyed over 10,000 people with endometriosis and interviewed health care practitioners and those with the condition about their experiences and found that:

- Average diagnosis times for endometriosis have not improved in over a decade—it still takes 8 years on average to get a diagnosis
- Prior to getting a diagnosis and with symptoms:
  - 58% visited their GP more than 10 times
  - 43% visited doctors in hospital over 5 times
  - 53% visited A&E
- Once diagnosed, only 19% know if they were seen in an endometriosis specialist centre
- 90% would have liked access to psychological support but were not offered this

To support those with endometriosis, the APPG has called on all governments in the UK to commit to a series of support measures for those with endometriosis including:

- Commitment to reduce average diagnosis times with a target of 4 years or less by 2025, and a year or less by 2030
- To ensure a baseline for endometriosis diagnosis, treatment and management by implementing the NICE Guideline on Endometriosis Treatment and Management (2017), adopted across the UK but not implemented
- Up to 10% of those with endometriosis will have the disease outside the pelvic cavity, yet the NICE Guideline only provides a care pathway for endometriosis within the pelvic cavity
- The APPG is calling for NICE to ensure that care pathways for all locations of endometriosis are developed and implemented, starting with thoracic endometriosis
- Investigation into the barriers faced in accessing care for those from Black, Asian and minority ethnic backgrounds, and ending the ethnicity and gender gaps in medical research
- Investment in research to find the cause of endometriosis; better treatment, management and diagnosis options; and, one day, a cure
- A commitment from all four nations to include compulsory menstrual wellbeing in the school curriculum so that young people recognize the warning signs of menstrual health conditions and know when to seek help. This is compulsory in schools in England from 2020 but is not UK wide

Sir David Amess MP, Chair of the APPG on Endometriosis, states:

> The report provides a stark picture of the reality of living with endometriosis, including the huge, life-long impact it may have on all aspects of life. It is not acceptable that endometriosis and its potentially debilitating and damaging symptoms are often ignored or not taken seriously—or downplayed as linked to the menstrual cycle and periods.
>
> All UK Governments must take the recommendations in this report seriously and act to ensure that everyone with endometriosis has a prompt diagnosis, along with access to the physical and mental health support they need to manage their condition.
>
> The APPG heard many accounts of people with endometriosis not having access to the specialist care they need. Only 19% of those who responded to the survey knew they were seen by a specialist centre, and 90% would have liked access to psychological support yet this was never offered.
>
> Our report highlights the urgent need for more research into the experiences and needs of those from LGBTQ+, Black, Asian and minority ethnic backgrounds. We must do more to understand the health inequalities and barriers for those from minority backgrounds in accessing the care they need.
>
> The APPG will not rest until tangible improvements are delivered to all those who suffer from this condition.

Implementing the recommendations in the report will reduce diagnosis time and ensure access to a minimum level of treatment and support for all those with endometriosis—saving on GP, hospital and A&E visits, as well as enabling those with the disease to live the productive lives they want.

The NICE Guideline produced in 2017 gives the baseline for care, but despite being adopted across the UK, it has not been implemented—it needs to be.

Commenting on the report, Emma Cox, CEO of Endometriosis UK, said:

> This report should be the final warning to Governments and the NHS that action must be taken on endometriosis. Implementing the recommendations in the report will reduce diagnosis time and ensure access to a minimum level of treatment and support for all those with endometriosis—saving on GP, hospital and A&E visits, as well as enabling those with the disease to live the productive lives they want.

She also said:

> *The average diagnosis time for endometriosis remains at 8 years—shockingly, it's not changed in a decade. Action must be taken to drive this down. The post code lottery of access to healthcare practitioners who specialise in endometriosis needs to end. Implementing effective processes within the NHS will help healthcare practitioners support diagnosis and get those with endometriosis symptoms to the right place, in hospitals with the right expertise, at the right time.*
>
> *Action is needed now, to ensure the next generation with endometriosis are not robbed of the future they deserve.*

ACTION BY WHO—CURRENT PRIORITIES (18)

The World Health Organization (WHO) has mentioned the following priorities related to endometriosis:

- Raising awareness about endometriosis among health care providers, women, men, adolescents, teachers and wider communities. Local, national and international information campaigns to educate the public and health care providers about normal and abnormal menstrual health and symptoms are needed
- Training all health care providers to improve their competency and skills to screen, diagnose, manage or refer patients with endometriosis. This can range from basic training of primary health care providers to recognize endometriosis to the advanced training of specialist surgeons and multidisciplinary teams
- Ensuring that primary health care plays a role in screening, identifying and providing basic pain management of endometriosis, in situations where gynaecologists or advanced multidisciplinary specialists are unavailable
- Advocating for health policies that ensure access to at least a minimum level of treatment and support for patients with endometriosis
- Setting up referral systems and care pathways consisting of well-linked primary health care centres and secondary and tertiary centres with advanced imaging, pharmacologic, surgical, fertility and multidisciplinary interventions
- Strengthening capacity of health systems to achieve early diagnosis and management of endometriosis by enhancing availability of equipment (e.g., ultrasound or magnetic resonance imaging) and

pharmaceuticals (e.g., nonsteroidal analgesics, combined oral contraceptives and progestin-based contraceptives)

- Increasing research on the pathogenesis, pathophysiology, natural progression, genetic and environmental risk factors, prognosis, disease classification, non-invasive diagnostic biomarkers, personalized treatments and other treatment paradigms, role of surgery, novel targeted therapeutics, curative therapies and preventive interventions in endometriosis (1,7)
- Accelerating collaborative global action to improve access to reproductive health care for women globally, including in low- and middle-income countries

WHO recognizes the importance of endometriosis and its impact on people's sexual and reproductive health, quality of life and overall wellbeing.

WHO aims to stimulate and support the adoption of effective policies and interventions to address endometriosis globally, especially in low- and middle-income countries.

WHO is partnering with multiple stakeholders, including academic institutions and other organizations that are actively involved in research, to identify effective models of endometriosis prevention, diagnosis, treatment and care.

WHO recognizes the importance of advocating for increased awareness, policies and services for endometriosis and collaborates with civil society and endometriosis patient support groups in this regard.

WHO is also collaborating with relevant stakeholders to facilitate and support the collection and analysis of country- and region-specific endometriosis prevalence data for decision-making.

KEY POINT SUMMARY

- Endometriosis poses a diagnostic dilemma in primary care settings, and uncertainty at initial consultations is common.
- Despite the prevalence and the severity of the condition, there remain many challenges in endometriosis care, with delayed diagnosis, a lack of patient-friendly diagnostics and a need for more targeted treatments.
- In the UK, work absenteeism and health care costs related to endometriosis cause economic losses of around £8.2 billon a year (direct treatment costs are comparable to those for type 2 diabetes and rheumatoid arthritis) (16).

- Improving diagnosis and non-invasive screening tools are among the top 10 research priorities for endometriosis in the UK (19).

REFERENCES

1. Zondervan KT, Becker CM, Missmer SA. Endometriosis. *N Engl J Med* 2020;382:1244–56.
2. Agarwal SK, Chapron C, Giudice LC, et al. Clinical diagnosis of endometriosis: A call to action. *Am J Obstet Gynecol* 2019;(4):354–64.
3. All Party Parliamentary Group on Endometriosis, Endometriosis UK. *Endometriosis in the UK: Time for change.* London: Endometriosis UK, 2020. www.endometriosis-uk.org/sites/default/files/files/Endometriosis%20 APPG%20Report%20Oct%202020.pdf (accessed 25 Aug 2023).
4. Ballard KD, Seaman HE, de Vries CS, et al. Can symptomatology help in the diagnosis of endometriosis? Findings from a national case-control study—Part 1. *BJOG* 2008;115:1382–91. doi:10.1111/j.1471-0528.2008.01878.x pmid:18715240 [CrossRef] [PubMed] [Web of Science] [Google Scholar]
5. Royal College of Obstetricians & Gynaecologists. Diagnostic Laparoscopy (Consent Advice No. 2). https://www.rcog.org.uk/guidance/browse-all-guidance/consent-advice/diagnostic-laparoscopy-consent-advice-no-2/
6. Pugsley Z, Ballard K. Management of endometriosis in general practice: The pathway to diagnosis. *Br J Gen Pract* 2007;57:470–6. pmid:17550672 [Abstract/FREE Full Text] [Google Scholar]
7. Soliman AM, Fuldeore M, Snabes MC. Factors associated with time to endometriosis diagnosis in the United States. *J Womens Health (Larchmt)* 2017;26:788–97. doi:10.1089/jwh.2016.6003 pmid:28440744 [CrossRef] [PubMed] [Google Scholar]
8. Sarıdoğan E. Endometriosis in teenagers. *Womens Health (Lond)* 2015; 11:705–9. doi:10.2217/whe.15.58 pmid:26315257 [CrossRef] [PubMed] [Google Scholar]
9. Prescott J, Farland LV, Tobias DK, et al. Endometriosis can double the risk of infertility in under 35s. A prospective cohort study of endometriosis and subsequent risk of infertility. *Hum Reprod* (2016);31(7):1475–82.
10. Nisenblat V, Bossuyt PMM, Shaikh R, et al. Blood biomarkers for the non-invasive diagnosis of endometriosis. *Cochrane Database Syst Rev* 2016;5:CD012179. doi:10.1002/14651858.CD012179 pmid:27132058 [CrossRef] [PubMed] [Google Scholar]
11. Nisenblat V, Bossuyt PMM, Farquhar C, et al. Imaging modalities for the non-invasive diagnosis of endometriosis. *Cochrane Database Syst Rev* 2016;2:CD009591. doi:10.1002/14651858.CD009591.pub2 pmid: 26919512 [CrossRef] [PubMed] [Google Scholar]
12. Hirsch M, Begum MR, Paniz É, et al. Diagnosis and management of endometriosis: A systematic review of international and national guidelines. *BJOG* 2018;125:556–64. doi:10.1111/1471-0528.14838 pmid:28755422 [CrossRef] [PubMed] [Google Scholar]
13. Gusovsky D. *Women suffering in silence: The endometriosis crisis.* https:// www.cnbc.com/2016/05/19.This-neglected-disease-is-a-hiddendrain-on-women's-success html
14. Sarıdoğan E. Endometriosis in teenagers. *Women's Health (Lond)* 2015; 11:705–9. doi:10.2217/whe.15.58 pmid:26315257 [CrossRef] [PubMed] [Google Scholar]

15. Culley L, Law C, Hudson N, et al. The social and psychological impact of endometriosis on women's lives: A critical narrative review. *Hum Reprod Update* 2013;19:625–39. doi:10.1093/humupd/dmt027 pmid:23884896 [CrossRef] [PubMed] [Web of Science] [Google Scholar]

16. Simoens S, Dunselman G, Dirksen C, et al. The burden of endometriosis: Costs and quality of life of women with endometriosis and treated in referral centres. *Hum Reprod* 2012;27:1292–9. doi:10.1093/humrep/des073 pmid:22422778 [CrossRef] [PubMed] [Web of Science] [Google Scholar]

17. Moss KM, Doust J, Homer H, et al. Delayed diagnosis of endometriosis disadvantages women in ART: A retrospective population linked data study. Hum Reprod2021;36:3074–82. doi:10.1093/humrep/deab216 pmid:34610108 [CrossRef] [PubMed] [Google Scholar]

18. World Health Organization (WHO). *International classification of diseases*, 11th Revision (ICD-11). Geneva: WHO 2018.

19. Horne AW, Saunders PTK, Abokhrais IM, et al. Endometriosis priority setting partnership steering group (appendix): Top ten endometriosis research priorities in the UK and Ireland. *Lancet* 2017;389:2191–2. doi:10.1016/S0140-6736(17)31344-2 pmid:28528751 [CrossRef] [PubMed] [Google Scholar]

FURTHER READING

All Party Parliamentary Group on Endometriosis, Endometriosis UK. *Endometriosis in the UK: Time for change.* London: Endometriosis UK, 2020. www.endometriosis-uk.org/sites/default/files/files/Endometriosis%20APPG%20Report%20Oct%202020.pdf (accessed 25 Aug 2023).

Primary Care Women's Health Forum. *10 top tips for endometriosis management in primary care.* Arlesey: PCWHF, 2021. pcwhf.co.uk/wp-content/uploads/2022/05/HLHH_Spring21_toptipsendo.pdf (accessed 20 Sep 2023).

Index

Note: Page numbers in *italics* indicate a figure and page numbers in **bold** indicate a table on the corresponding page.